BEAUTIFUL SKIN

BEAUTIFUL SKIN

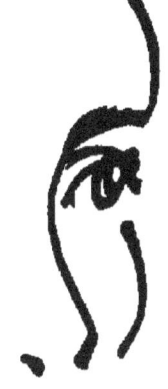

CONSUMER GUIDE TO COSMETIC BOTOX®
TREATMENT AND SKIN CARE

Joseph A. Mauriello, Jr, MD

Writers Club Press
New York Lincoln Shanghai

Beautiful Skin
Consumer Guide to Cosmetic Botox® Treatment and Skin Care

Writers Club Press
an imprint of iUniverse, Inc.

For information address:
iUniverse
2021 Pine Lake Road, Suite 100
Lincoln, NE 68512
www.iuniverse.com

Please note that the information contained in this book is educational. It does intend to constitute a second opinion or to create a physician-patient relationship. Also, it is not intended to violate any pre-existing physician-patient relationship.

ISBN: 0-595-25423-3

Printed in the United States of America

This book is dedicated to my wife, Marilyn, and to all people whose "Beautiful Eyes and Skin" are only matched by the goodness of their hearts.

CONTENTS

PREFACE

Purpose of Cosmetic Botox® Treatments

- *Do you have frown lines between your eyebrows and do people sometimes ask you why are you frowning?*

- *Do you have squint lines in the corner of your eyes?*

- *Are your lips thin, and do you notice lipstick lines that smear your lipstick?*

COSMETIC BOTOX® treatments are performed in the office, have no down time, and enhance appearance. Various medical societies, including the American Academy of Cosmetic Surgery, recognize the procedure as the most common cosmetic procedure.

Unwanted facial lines are temporarily erased or reduced after a simple office treatment. Evaluation and treatment are performed during the same visit. The patient drives to the office and drives away a few minutes later.

The effects are noted gradually over the next 7 to 14 days. The individual's appearance and facial expression are not changed when the injections are performed to produce a nondistorted, subtle result. The injections should not create a plastic, expressionless appearance, but, instead, they restore a youthful refreshed appearance.

The art of using Botox is to minimize the dose and selectively treat specific unwanted lines. The treatment should be individualized for each patient since each patient has a different pattern of wrinkles and preferences to remove only certain unwanted facial lines.

The July 31th, 2000, "Marketplace Section" of the Wall Street Journal, contains a report of an investment banker who was laid off and unable to convert interviews into job offers. The executive recruiter indicated that his resume was excellent but that he had an "angry" appearance. Botox A not only took care of the deep lines on the banker's foreheads but he soon found a job. The same article quotes a recent online survey by the American Society of Plastic Surgeons. This survey discovered that 12% of patients who responded requested Botox to improve a "severe/angry facial expression."

Botox injections enhance cosmetic eyelid surgery
Botox injections are not a substitute for cosmetic eyelid surgery that removes excess skin overhanging the upper eyelid crease or fat bulges surrounding the upper and lower eyelids. Only surgery may remove loose, baggy, and inelastic skin.

Botox injections complement cosmetic eyelid surgery by reducing crow's feet in the corner of the eyes and smoothing skin around the eyes.

After performing several thousand cosmetic Botox® injections as well as functional Botox injections for eyelid spasms and over 6000 eyelid surgeries, Dr. Mauriello has found that many patients are enthusiastic about the results and virtually all patients are extremely satisfied.

Importance of skin care

A skin care regimen provided by a physician prevents further photoaging of the skin. Skin care improves the texture and thickness of the skin and enhances the results of the cosmetic Botox injections and cosmetic eyelid surgery. Skin care requires a daily regimen. Self-neutralizing skin peels have less down time than more aggressive peels and produce gradual but definite results over time.

Goals of the book

This book is written for individuals who are considering cosmetic Botox injections and wish to be educated. Its main goal is to make information available to you, the consumer. It is written so that you will then be able to review the various sections of the book at your leisure. The book, therefore, complements a relatively short surgical consultation and should completely replace information obtained from a friend who may have undergone previous cosmetic surgery. Each patient has different concerns and responds uniquely to any cosmetic procedure including Botox injections. Although no reading material replaces the intimacy and one-on-one benefits of a pre-surgical consultation, this book helps you determine whether you are a candidate for cosmetic Botox office injections by providing you with pertinent questions to ask the surgeon during the consultation.

Outline of book

This book helps you to:

- determine whether you are a candidate for Botox office injections
- select a surgeon
- examine actual patient results before and after Botox treatment
- implement a personal skin care regimen with the assistance of your physician

A glossary of terms is available to the reader at the end of the text.

Types of doctors who perform Botox treatments

Various types of physicians perform cosmetic Botox treatment and these include plastic surgeons, dermatologists, facial plastic surgeons, otolaryngologists with specialized training in facial plastic surgery, and ophthalmologists. This book is written by an oculoplastic surgeon, an ophthalmologist specializing in eyelid surgery. In any event, the individual should select a physician who has concentrated his efforts on cosmetic procedures.

Autobiographical note

Joseph A. Mauriello, Jr, MD is one of a handful of ophthalmologists in New Jersey who specializes in ophthalmic plastic and reconstructive (oculoplastic) surgery that involves eyelid as well as tear duct, socket, or orbital surgery. He is one of approximately 400 physicians nationally who is a member of the American Society of Ophthalmic Plastic and Reconstructive Surgery. Dr. Mauriello, Director of Oculoplastic Surgery at UMD-NJ Medical School at Newark from 1983 to 1998, was the first ophthalmologist to dedicate his entire medical practice to

Oculoplastic surgery in New Jersey. He is, therefore, in a unique position to educate the patient.

Since moving his office to Summit, NJ in 1998, he has dedicated a large portion of his practice to cosmetic eyelid surgery and office Botox injections.

About Dr. Mauriello's Training After completing medical school training at UMD—New Jersey Medical School, Newark, NJ and an ophthalmology residency at New York University Medical Center, Dr. Mauriello received a two-year training grant from the National Eye Institute for a Fellowship in ophthalmic pathology at the Armed Forces Institute of Pathology (AFIP). The AFIP has 39 branches and serves as a consultative pathology center for the armed forces but also for civilian pathologists. The world-renown Ophthalmic Pathology branch is a referral center for diagnosing tissue specimens from the eye, eyelids, orbit, and lacrimal system. During his training at the AFIP, he also studied dermatopathology. This training serves as a basis for much of the cosmetic skin care performed in his office.

After completing the two-year fellowship at the AFIP in 1982, Dr. Mauriello trained in ophthalmic plastic and reconstructive surgery (oculoplastic surgery) at Wills Eye Hospital in Philadelphia. Dr. Mauriello was honored to receive an additional one-year grant awarded by the Heed Ophthalmic Foundation in Chicago. This foundation supports promising young investigators who pursue advanced subspecialty training in ophthalmology.

While there are no subspecialty boards in ophthalmology or oculoplastic surgery, the American Society of Ophthalmic

Plastic and Reconstructive Surgery elects candidates as Fellows. Such fellows complete four years of medical school. After receiving their doctor of medicine degree, they then complete a one-year approved internship that usually includes surgical training. A three- or four-year residency in ophthalmology is completed and requirements for Board Certification by the American Board of Ophthalmology are met. In addition, candidates must complete an approved fellowship in ophthalmic plastic and reconstructive surgery and write a thesis that is approved by the Thesis Committee. They must also pass written and oral examinations.

About Dr. Mauriello's Experience Dr. Mauriello was also honored to be selected as one of the BEST DOCTORS OF AMERICA (1998) according to the input of 35,000 physicians both locally and nationally in a two year survey by Woodward/White. The Best Doctors in American is published annually in *New Jersey Magazine, Town and Country, and other periodicals.* He was again honored to be selected in the 2000-2001 listing of **BEST DOCTORS, Inc (BESTDOCTORS.COM)** He received the American Academy of Ophthalmology *Honor Award* in 1991 for his scientific and teaching contributions to the Academy. He has published with over 70 original articles in peer-reviewed journals and, in addition, published 30 chapters in scientific books.

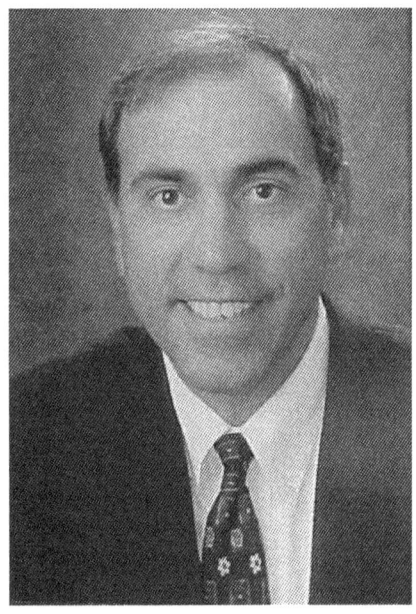

Dr. Mauriello was one of the first physician to use Botox in the New York metropolitan area in 1983. An original investigator in the National Institute of Health's study entitled Botulinum Toxin in the Treatment of Benign Essential Blepharospasm from 1983-1989, he was also a consultant to the Committee of Ophthalmic Procedures Assessment of the American Academy of Ophthalmology from 1985-89. He has been invited to the Speaker's Bureau of Allergan (distributors of Botox) Pharmaceutical (Irvine, California) since 1997. He served as a Reviewer of the American Academy of Neurology's Therapeutics Assessment Subcommittee on Botulinum toxin therapy in 1999, and participated in the combined NIH-National Blepharospasm Foundation Brainstorming Session in Washington, DC in late 2000.

Dr. Mauriello was honored to serve as Chairman of the Thesis Committee in the American Society of Ophthalmic Plastic and Reconstructive Surgery (ASOPRS) in 2002. This committee evaluates candidates' theses for membership in ASOPRS. Dr. Mauriello has also served on the Education Committee of the American Society of Ophthalmic Plastic and Reconstructive Surgery (ASOPRS) for over a decade. He has composed questions for the written examination for the society and has acted as an oral examiner for prospective candidates' theses prior to their acceptance into the Society.

Dr. Mauriello's books, *Beautiful Eyes Consumer's Guide to Cosmetic Eyelid Surgery*, and *Beautiful Skin*, are available at **www.iuniverse.com**, amazon.com, and bn.com (Barnes and Noble).

It answers all the consumer's questions about cosmetic eyelid surgery including whether you are a candidate for surgery and how to choose a surgeon. Patient testimonials provide practical information from the patient's viewpoint.

Dr. Mauriello has a unique practice that consists almost exclusively of eyelid surgery. In addition, he has a vast experience treating patients with Botox, since 1983.

Dr. Mauriello was honored to be elected to the international Orbital Society in 1994, a group of 25 members, and to serve as a reviewer for many of the major ophthalmologic journals. Finally, he was invited to serve on the Medical Advisory Board of the American Society of Ocularists in 2000.

Dr. Mauriello has presented over 100 papers at national meetings and has been selected for panels on national symposia throughout his career. He completed the editing of his second major medical textbook concerning eyelid and lacrimal surgery. The book is over 600 pages and contains a section dedicated to cosmetic forehead, eyelid, and midfacial cosmetic surgery. Its unique format includes expert commentary by prominent specialists in oculoplastic surgery, dermatology, plastic surgery, and otolaryngology who review and critique specific chapters. Butterworth Heineman, the international medical publisher in Boston (presently part of Elsevier Science, Inc), published the text in the summer of 2000. Dr. Mauriello's first textbook, *Management of Orbital and Ocular Adnexal Tumors and Inflammation*s, was co-authored with Dr. Joseph C. Flanagan, who is Director of Oculoplastic Surgery, at Wills Eye Hospital, Philadelphia, Pa.

Dr. Mauriello is presently working on a third major textbook, *Techniques of Cosmetic (Restorative) Eyelid Surgery:* **A Case Study Approach,** to be published by Lippincott Williams and Wilkins, Philadelphia, PA. This book considers subtle nuances of cosmetic eyelid surgery that avoid an abnormally pulled or operated facial appearance.

He was honored to be elected a fellow member of the American Academy of Cosmetic Surgery in 2001.

Dr. Mauriello's training and background are unique and he feels fortunate to be able to practice a distinct and unique subspecialty that includes cosmetic eyelid surgery and Botox injections. The greatest satisfaction is derived from helping others in this practice.

Joseph A. Mauriello, Jr, MD
Ophthalmic Plastic and Reconstructive Surgery
Fellow member, American Society of Ophthalmic Plastic and Reconstructive Surgery
Fellow member, American Academy of Cosmetic Surgery
Fellow, American Academy of Ophthalmology

Cosmetic Eyelid and Facial Rejuvenation Centers

Medical Arts Center	*Brook 35 Park*
33 Overlook Road, Suite 104	*2130 Highway 35, Suite 115*
Summit, NJ 07901	*Sea Girt, NJ 08750*
908-608-1200	*732—449-3299*

URL: EYELIDMD.NET

ACKNOWLEDGEMENTS

The author wishes to acknowledge all patients who allowed themselves to be photographed and included in this book.

CHAPTER 1

WHAT IS BOTOX AND HOW DOES IT WORK?

History of Botox®
Allergan's BOTOX® product was approved by the FDA for clinical use in 1989, and has a proven track record for the treatment of strabismus (crossed eyes) and blepharospasm (involuntary eyelid spasms). In December, 2000, Botox® was also approved for the treatment of abnormal head position and neck pain associated with cervical dystonia. Botox® Cosmetic was approved for the treatment of glabellar (between the eyebrows) frown and scowl lines in Canada in April, 2001 and in the United States in April, 2002.

Medical Uses of Botox
BOTOX® therapy is approved in 70 countries for a broad range of conditions. It is currently being investigated in the U.S. for the treatment of many different medical conditions:

- hyperhidrosis (excessive sweating)
- post-stroke muscle spasticity
- juvenile cerebral palsy

- spasticity including back spasm
- pain and headache including myofascial pain
- management of occupational dystonia (involuntary movement)
- writer's cramp
- temporomandibular disorders
- gastrointestinal disease
- urologic disorders
- tremors
- tics
- cosmetic uses

How does Botox work?

Botox blocks the nerve impulses that cause a voluntary skeletal muscle to contract. Botox ® is, therefore, called a "neurotoxin." Botox ® binds to special sites at terminals where the nerve and muscle interface. These terminals are known as motor nerve terminals. Specifically, Botox ® blocks the release of a chemical that causes the muscle to contract. The chemical, known as a neurotransmitter, is called "acetylcholine." Actually, Botox, the neurotoxin, cleaves to a special protein, the so-called "SNAP-25 protein" that is necessary for the release of the acetylcholine. Without the release of the acetylcholine, the muscle affected by the particular nerve terminal is unable to contract. Botox does not inactivate every tiny muscle fiber and, therefore, does not generally lead to complete loss of muscle function. The effect of Botox is temporary and eventually after 3 to 6 months the muscle contracts.

There are several types of botulinum toxin in nature. Different strains of the bacterium, *Clostridium botulinum,* are used in the preparation of each type of botulinum toxin. Only types A and B are commercially available. Type A is in Botox ® and Dysport® by Inamed. Type B is Myobloc®, made by Elan Pharmaceutical. One unit of Botox ® or Botox ® cosmetic is approximately equivalent to 3-5 Dysport® units and 50-150 Myobloc® units. Allergan's new formulation of Botox® is the same formulation as the original. However, the new formulation produced since 1997 has a higher specific potency. The improved bulk toxin reduces the neurotoxin protein utilized to deliver the same 100 units to 20% of original. This new formulation replaces original Botox® and, therefore, the development of antibodies that inactivate that drugs is reduced.

What is Botox ® Cosmetic?
Botox (R) Cosmetic (Botulinum Toxin Type A) is a purified Neurotoxin Complex. It is a sterile vacuum-dried purified botulinum toxin type A, produced from a strain of bacterium, *Clostridium botulinum* type A. The bacterium is grown in a specific culture. The culture is then purified and the resulting complex is dissolved in a sterile sodium chloride solution that contains human albumin and is sterile filtered. The drug is received in the physician's office in its frozen state in a vial that is kept frozen.

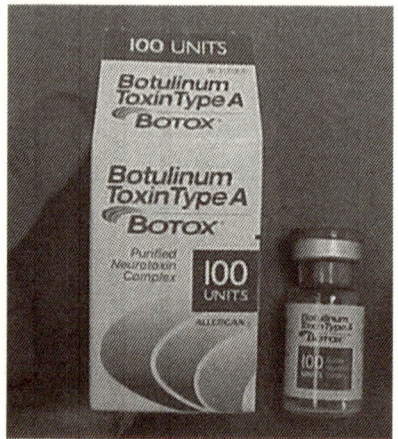

Note that the precipitated Botox® is at the bottom of the vial as shown by the arrow. Each Botox ® vial contains 100 units while each Dysport® vial contains 500 units (Dysport® is not approved for use in the United States as of 11-1-02). Myobloc® vials contain 2500 units per ½ ml, 5000 units per 1ml and 10,000 units per 2 ml. The number of units per vial are summized in the Table below.

Drug	units per vial	volume cc per vial
Botox ®	100 units	Dilute with usually 1 to 4 cc's for cosmetic facial use
Dysport®	500 units	Dilute as necessary
Myobloc®	5000 units per ml	Premixed

The day the Botox® is used, the physician reconstitutes the contents of the frozen vial to the desired concentration. Allergan recommends that the vial be used within four hours, since the reconstituted solution does not contain preservatives. It is estimated that the reconstituted drug loses minimal potency over two weeks if kept refrigerated. There are concerns of sterility once reconstituted, since the reconstituted form contains no preservatives. It is this office's policy to use the vial on the day it is opened. The vial is considered single-use, but it has been used in a sterile fashion for more than one patient and any residual is discarded that day.

Why do wrinkles form?
As skin becomes less elastic over time, repeated muscle frowning may create visible lines and wrinkles. Even inadvertent squinting due to light sensitivity may exacerbate the problem. Wrinkles result from sun damage and aging that decrease skin elasticity and lead to loss of the ground substance or matrix of the skin. Skin laxity that is not induced by underlying muscle contraction will not improve with Botox. It is important for a physician to analyze the cause of your wrinkles. Skin care augments the effects of cosmetic Botox treatment.

How does Botox improve my wrinkles?
By weakening muscles, the overlying skin lines produced by the muscle contractions are less pronounced.

Are there other drugs similar to Botox that may be used for wrinkle treatment?
Myobloc®, botulinum toxin Type B, is made by Elan Pharmaceutical. It has only been approved by the FDA for cervical dystonia

(rigidity and muscular spasms of the neck). Therefore, use of Myobloc® to reduce wrinkles is an off-label use.

Botox® is only drug approved by the FDA as of 2002 to treat frown lines between the eyebrows at this time. Injection of other sites in the face are considered "off-label" uses. As of 2002, Dysport, botulinum toxin type A, is available in Europe and is presently in its clinical testing stages for FDA approval in the US. It will be marketed by Inamed when it becomes available.

Is Botox a poison?

Botox is the same chemical that causes botulism. This condition causes death by weakening the muscles of respiration. There is an antidote for botulism which will only diminish the effect of new Botox that is subsequently given. It will not neutralize any drug that has already attached to the muscle.

> *Dr. Mauriello's Comments: Dr. Mauriello has performed over 6000 Botox injections in patients in the eyelid, facial, and neck tissues since 1983. Dr. Mauriello has not had to consider any antidotal treatment for any of his patients to date.*

Any drug is potentially a poison if given in sufficient dose. Botulinum toxin was only known for its toxic effects until its therapeutic effects were appreciated and developed by Dr. Alan Scott, an ophthalmologist at Pacific Medical Center in the late 1970's. He developed the drug to treat crossed eyes in children and adults. Every drug has an LD-50. The LD-50 is the dose of a drug that given in an experimental system, and will cause 50% of mice that are injected with a given dose to die. It is estimated that 40 vials of Botox, each of which contains 100 units, are toxic to humans. Generally, one-quarter to one-third of a vial is injected in the facial regions for cosmetic indications.

The injections of Botox in the desired doses represent extremely small quantities of the drug and the only way Botox will cause a problem is if the injection is given in a muscle that has a critical function or an inadvertent overdose is given. In order to have continued therapeutic effect, Botox needs to be re-injected at certain intervals because its effect wears off at the site it is injected.

Does the drug affect my whole body?
The drug is injected at the site where its effects are desired. Minute amounts are not detectable in the blood when given in doses in the therapeutic range. Nonetheless, when sensitive studies called single fiber electromyography are performed to measure minute muscle activity, the effects of the drug are measurable at sites distant from the injection.

Are there potential unreported or unknown side-effects?
There is always the extremely rare risk of an unknown side-effect with any drug. The drug has been FDA approved for other uses since 1988.

Dr. Mauriello has treated several hundred patients with this drug since 1983. Some patients have received as many 30 injections over the years since the effects are temporary and repeat injections are necessary. As a result, he has personally given over 6000 injections and has noted only minimal side effects.

What are possible side-effects?
The possible side effects are listed below.

Pain at injection site: The most common side-effect is mild pain on injection which dissipates almost immediately after the injection is given. There in no pain after the procedure and no medication is required.

Mild Bruising: There may be slight bruising at the site or even a small hematoma or collection of blood under the skin with minimal discomfort. As with any bruise, this problem resolves itself over 7 to14 days and may be treated, if desired, with ice the first 48 hours four times a day for 5 minutes (ice may be placed in a Ziploc bag). Make-up may be used to conceal any discoloration.

Headache, respiratory infection, Flu syndrome, and nausea: In clinical trials conducted by Allergan, Inc., the most frequently reported adverse events were studied. In this study, patients received either Botox or a placebo (a pseudo-drug without any pharmacologic effect). Patients reported the following side-effects without knowledge of what they had taken (the investigators had no knowledge as well):

	Botox Treated Group	Placebo (nontreated group)
Headache	13.3%	17.7%
Respiratory infection	3.5%	3.8%
Blepharoptosis		
Temporary eyelid droop	3.2%	0%
Nausea	3.0%	2.3%
Flu syndrome	2.0%	1.5%

Note that the incidence of all side-effects, except for the temporary eyelid droop, occurred significantly in the placebo group as well as the Botox group.

In Dr. Mauriello's experience, even the "most common" side-effects are uncommon.

Ptosis (drooping) of the Upper Lid: Ptosis of the upper lid is possible but extremely rare. In treating facial lines in the forehead, your physician will selectively weaken the muscles that close the eyes. These latter muscles are anatomically close to the muscles that elevate the lid, and the potential to weaken the eyelid elevators exists.

Dr. Mauriello's comments regarding ptosis (drooping of the upper lid) after Botox injections: *Dr. Mauriello has observed two cases of ptosis after several hundred Botox injections for cosmetic reasons. He examined a patient who was referred to him by a plastic surgeon. This patient developed ptosis subsequent to treatment elsewhere. Like virtually all side-effects, the ptosis subsequently resolved. The second patient had a pre-existing drooping lid. The technique of injection should virtually eliminate this rare, transient complication of Botox ® Cosmetic.*

BOTOX® COSMETIC should not be used in the presence of infection at the proposed injection site(s).

Botox Allergy Extremely Rare: As with any drug, serious allergic reaction may occur that necessitates treatment. Dr. Mauriello has encountered two patients with allergic reactions. Should a rash develop, the physician should be called. However, should a full-blown allergy (known as an anaphylactic reaction) including tightness of the throat and shortness of breath develop, emergency treatment is warranted.

In Dr. Mauriello's two patients with allergic reactions, both patients experienced reactions to the experimental form of Botulinum toxin, type A, before it was approved by the FDA. One developed a skin rash when injected at two separate times, and the other developed a skin rash and a tightness of the throat. In both instances, the drug was no longer given.

Avoid Botox in pregnancy: Botox should not be used during pregnancy, since no testing has established its safety during pregnancy.

Muscle weakness: Systemic weakness or muscle paralysis may occur. Difficulty swallowing has occurred rarely after treatment of the neck muscles. The treatment of the neck should not usually exceed more than 30 units at one time.

Possible Drug Interactions: Botox should be used extremely judiciously in conjunction with certain drugs that interfere with neuromuscular activity. The drugs include antibiotics such as amino-glycosides, curare, lincosamides, polymyxin antibiotics, quinidine, magnesium sulfate, anticholinesterases, and succinylcholine. The physician who treats you will obtain a complete medical history that includes the history of medications you are talking. Always check with your physician if you have any concerns. In this regard, the drug should be used cautiously in any patient with a neuromuscular disease, including rare diseases such as myasthenia gravis.

Dr. Mauriello has not experienced a drug interaction in his practice.

Other possible Side-effects: Since Botox is produced and contains human albumin, there is an extremely remote risk of viral disease transmission. This risk is minimized by donor screening and the manufacturing processes. No documented case of Creutzfeld Jakob ("Mad Cow Disease") disease has been reported to date.

Antidote for overdose: As stated above, virtually every drug overdose may be treated. In the case of Botox, an antidote is available should an overdose or misinjection be given to a patient. The antidote prevents additional muscle weakness but will not influence muscle weakness that has already occurred.

> **Dr. Mauriello's commentary:** *Dr. Mauriello has never had to treat a patient with an overdose of Botox®. He finds it safest to use the drug discretely and incrementally over several visits to obtain the desired result. In this way, overdose is avoided. When the patient returns for retreatment several months later, the cumulative dose is injected in one treatment session.*

When large doses are given in the neck region, a single patient experienced problems with swallowing known as dysphagia. For this reason, low doses are given in the neck area not to exceed 30 to 40 units (*Carruthers J, Carruthers A: Practical cosmetic BOTOX techniques. J Cutaneous Med Surg 3:55-59, 1999 (suppl 4)*).

If some Botox is good, is more better?: The simple answer is "no." For any cosmetic procedure, it is far better to achieve a "good" response than to have a complication. The tolerance for problems with cosmetic surgery is very low.

> *Dr. Mauriello's commentary: A patient came into Dr. Mauriello's office and stated that she wanted to get the greatest effect from Botox. She requested additional injections after she was already treated in the incremental fashion outlined above. Increasing the dose of Botox once the optimum dose for any given patient is established is against Dr. Mauriello's philosophy. Adding more Botox will only increase the risks of additional side-effects. Certainly, increasing the Botox will not increase its duration of 3 to 6 months. If two aspirins relieve a headache, ten aspirins may cause side-effects.*

Dr. Mauriello's Treatment Philosophy: Dr. Mauriello attempts to determine the optimum dose for a specific area of the face in any given patient over two or three treatment sessions. Initial treatment requires injection of specific muscle groups to determine the effects of the Botox® on the particular individual receiving treatment. Photographic documentation allows Dr. Mauriello to analyze the effects of each treatment. Once that optimal dose is determined, reinjections at the same dose level are given in a single future office visit with fairly predictable results. Dr. Mauriello encourages patients to wait 4 months between cosmetic injections. Repeat injections at short intervals are not advisable over time, and, although rarely, may lead to tolerance to the drug so that it does not work.

How effective is Botox® Cosmetic in Reducing wrinkles?
Allergan performed studies to determine the efficacy of Botox in treated the glabellar frown lines between the eyebrows above the nose.

The following data are provided by Allergan Pharmaceuticals, 2525 Dupont Drive, Irvine,California 92612 through a subsidiary, Allergan Pharmaceuticals, Ireland Ltd.). In the Allergan-funded studies, frown lines were judged as "none," "mild," "moderate," or "severe." The ratings were performed 30 days after treatment. The response to the Botox was judged on a scale of "+4 to –4," where "+4" was considered complete improvement, and "–4" was considered "very marked worsening" or about 100% worse or greater. A moderate improvement was "+2 "(about 50%).

The participants in the study ranged in age from 22 to 78 years with a mean age of 46 years. Woman predominated and represented 81.9% of the study while 83.8% were white. Facial wrinkles were reduced up to 120 days.

The results of the Allergan sponsored study are summarized below:

Investigator's assessment	Severity of lines judged as "mild or none"
Day 7 after Botox	73.8%
Day 30	80.2%
Day 60	70.2%
Day 90	47.6%
Day 120	25.3%

Patient's or Subject's assessment

Day 7	82.5%
Day 30	89.4%
Day 60	81.9%
Day 90	63%
Day 120	39%

As the Allergan data show, the patients experienced a subjective sense of a better response to the wrinkle treatment than did the investigators' assessment. During the 12-month study, 537 patients were evaluated. Four hundred and five patients obtained Botox ® injections, and 132 received a placebo. The study was double-blind in that neither the patients nor the investigating physicians were aware of which patients received Botox and which received the placebo. The placebo group did not receive any Botox. During the first 8 months of the study, the maximum response rate occurred at day 30 after treatment. The investigators found that 80.2% of the subjects treated with BOTOX® COSMETIC, versus 3.0% of those subjects treated with placebo, responded to treatment. The criterion for response was reduction in the severity of glabellar lines at maximum frown. In addition, a significant improvement in brow furrow appearance (rated by the subject's self-assessment) also occurred in 89.4% of those treated with BOTOX® COSMETIC, and only 6.8% of the placebo group.

More marked improvement of 84.6% was experienced by patients less than 50 years of age. Marked improvement was 70.4% in patients aged 50 to 65, and 39.1% in patients over 65 years of age.

How long does it take for Botox to have an effect?

It generally takes 7 to 10 days. Patients may experience some relief almost immediately. In the majority of patients, the drug takes effect in 10 to 14 days. Each patient has a biologic response unique to his or her system. The results tend to be consistent for any given patient. In other words, if the drug starts working in 4 days, it will generally have an effect in 4 days on subsequent treatments.

How long does Botox work?

For any given patient, it usually lasts 3 to 6 months. If a patient has a result that lasts 6 months, that patient will generally experience the same result on subsequent treatments. Again, Dr. Mauriello recommends a return for retreatment after at least 4 months.

How does Botox help patients with involuntary eyelids spasms? Dr. Mauriello's interest is Botox is summarized by a list of publications and presentations below:

During Dr. Mauriello's fellowship in Oculoplastic Surgery at Will's Eye Hospital in 1982, patients with blepharospasm were often prescribed dark glasses and oral medications both of which provided little relief. The patients with severe blepharospasm were offered frontalis suspension (surgical suspension of the eyelids to the eyebrows) to help break the eyelid spasms. All patients with hemifacial spasm were considered possible candidates for neurosurgery, since oral pharmacologic agents rarely controlled the problem. Hemifacial spasm consists on spasm on one side of the face and is most commonly due to a tortuous vessel at the brainstem level that impinges on the seventh nerve that supplies one side of the face.

> *Dr. Mauriello visited Alan Scott, MD (Pacific Medical Center, San Francisco, California) who demonstrated the effectiveness of botulinum toxin in the treatment of blepharospasm and hemifacial spasm. Dr. Mauriello was one of the first physicians to bring this treatment to the New York metropolitan area in 1983.*

Dr. Mauriello was honored to be one of the original investigators of the National Institute of Health's study entitled Botulinum Toxin in the Treatment of Benign Essential Blepharospasm. This multicenter national center study was conducted from 1983-1989 and was headed by Dr. Scott. Dr. Mauriello was selected to act as a consultant to the Committee of Ophthalmic Procedures Assessment of the American Academy of Ophthalmology from 1985-89 to evaluate the effectiveness of botulinum toxin, type A, when the toxin was in its experimental stage.

Dr. Mauriello was invited to the Speaker's Bureau of Allergan Pharmaceutical (Irvine, California) in 1997. Since early 2000, he has been honored to serve as a Reviewer of the American Academy of Neurology's Therapeutics Assessment Subcommittee on Botulinum toxin therapy. He served on the Board of Medical Advisors of the Northern New Jersey Chapter of the national Benign Essential Blepharospasm Research Foundation from 1985-88.

Dr. Mauriello's papers and presentations that related to botulinum toxin are outlined below:

PUBLICATIONS

Mauriello JA. Blepharospasm, Meige syndrome, and hemi-facial spasm: treatment with botulinum toxin. *Neurology* 35: 1949-1500, 1985.

Mauriello, JA, Coniaris, Haupt E. Use of botulinum toxin in the treatment of one hundred patients with facial dyskinesias. *Ophthalmology* 94:976-79, 1987.

Mauriello JA, Aljian JA. Natural history of the treatment of facial dyskinesias with botulinum toxin: A study of 50 consecutive patients over 7 years. *British Journal Ophthalmology* 75:737-739, 1991.

Mauriello JA et al. Treatment profile of 239 patients with blepharospasm and Meige syndrome over 11 years. *British Journal Ophthalmology* 80:1073-75, 1996.

The long-term treatment preferences of 239 patients with blepharospasm and Meige syndrome were studied. , 202 patients (72.1%) continued treatment with botulinum toxin, type A. Five patients had remission of their disease. This study demonstrated the long-term acceptance of botulinum toxin by a large cohort of patients.

Mauriello JA et al. Treatment choices of 119 patients with hemi-facial spasm over 11 years. *Clinical Neurology and Neurosurgery* 98:213-6, 1996.

This study demonstrated the long-term acceptance of botulinum toxin type A and the treatment of choice for hemifacial spasm. Five of the 119 patients had unexplained spontaneous resolution of their condition after botulinum toxin, type A, treatment.

Mauriello et al. Drug associated dyskinesias—a study of 238 patients. *Neuro-ophthalmology* 18:153-7, 1998.

It is difficult to prove that any drug causes blepharospasm. However, certain medications including antidepressants and anti-psychotic medications are associated with blepharospasm. After cessation of the presumed offending anti-psychotic medication, it may take years for the effect on eyelid spasms to dissipate.

Mauriello et al. Long-term enhancement of botulinum toxin injections by upper eyelid surgery in 14 patients with facial dyskinesias. *Archives Otolaryngology-Head and Neck Surgery* 125: 627-31, 1999.

In patients with a partial response response to botulinum toxin, type A, and in other patients with excess skin over-hanging the upper eyelid margin, limited myectomy (removal of muscle in the upper lid) and even upper lid blepharoplasty with repair of ptosis (drooping upper eyelid) alone without myectomy significantly improved both the duration and response to botulinum toxin injections. All patients would opt for surgery again. All had the side benefit of improved cosmesis.

Mauriello JA. Treatment of benign essential blepharospasm and hemifacial spasm: a preliminary study of 68 patients. In: *Advances in Ophthalmic Plastic Surgery* (Volume 4), Smith B and Bosniak S (eds); Pergammon Press, NY, NY, 1985, pp 283-289.

Mauriello et al. Oculinum therapy: its use in neuro-ophthalmology (Treatment of Facial Dyskinesia) in *Neuro-ophthalmological disorders*, Tusa R, Newman SA (ed); Marcel Dekker, 1994, 451-77.

Mauriello JA. Editorial commentary: Causes and treatment of blepharospasm: botulinum toxin, limited myectomy, and pharmacologic therapy on Surgical management of essential blepharospasm, Patel BCK, Anderson Rl. Chapter 8, 197-204 in *Unfavorable Results of Eyelid and Lacrimal Surgery Prevention and Management* Mauriello JA (ed); Butterworth Heinemann, Boston, MA, 2000.

Mauriello JA. Role of Botulinum Toxin Type A (BTX-A) (Botoxâ) in the Management of Blepharospasm and Hemifacial Spasm. *Scientific and Therapeutic Aspects of Botulinum Toxin*, ed. Brin M, Lippincott, Williams, & Wilkins, Philadelphia, Pa 2001.

INVITED SCIENTIFIC PRESENTATIONS (partial list)
Mauriello JA: Essential blepharospasm: a new treatment. New Jersey Academy of Ophthalmology, Fall, 1983.

Mauriello JA: Treatment of essential blepharospasm with botulinum toxin. NJ Academy of Ophthalmology, Ophthalmic Allied Health Symposium, Parsippany, NJ, October 10, 1984

Mauriello, JA: Treatment of essential blepharospasm. Channel 13 PBS, WNET, "Innovations," Newark, NJ, May 3 and May 6, 1984.

Mauriello JA: Treatment of Essential blepharospasm, Northern NJ Chapter of National Blepharospasm Foundation, St. Barnabas Medical Center, Livingston, NJ, May 1984.

Mauriello JA: Blepharospasm, NY Chapter of National Blepharospasm Foundation, Long Island Jewish Medical Center, NY, January 27, 1985.

Mauriello JA, Treatment of facial dyskinesias with botulinum toxin. Westchester County Medical Society, Valhalla, NY, April 30, 1985.

Mauriello JA: Treatment of blepharospasm with botulinum toxin. Grand Rounds, Department of Neurology, Rutgers Medical School, New Brunswick, NJ, March 23, 1985.

Wagner RS and Mauriello JA: The use of botulinum toxin for the treatment of strabismus and blepharospasm. Mediprecis 2:44-5, 1986.

Mauriello JA: Update on the treatment of blepharospasm with botulinum toxin. New Jersey Academy of Ophthalmology, Ophthalmic Allied Health Symposium, Long Branch, NJ, December 1, 1993.

Mauriello JA: Enhancement of botulinum toxin injections by upper eyelid surgery in the treatment of a cohort of 358 patients with facial dyskinesias. American Academy of Ophthalmology, fall, 1997.

Mauriello JA: Treatment of Blepharospasm and hemifacial spasm with botulinum toxin, International Symposium on Movement Disorders, Orlando, Florida, November 18,1999.

Mauriello JA: Surgical Management of blepharospasm, Beth Israel Medical Center, NY, NY, April 17, 1999.

Mauriello JA: Drug induced blepharospasm, Benign Essential Blepharospasm Research Foundation and the National Institute of Neurological Disorders, Bethesda, Maryland, November 17 and 17, 2000.

Mauriello JA: Surgical Treatment of Blepharospasm, Benign Essential Blepharospasm Research Foundation, Overlook Hospital, Summit, NJ, September 28, 2002.

CHAPTER 2

AM I A CANDIDATE FOR BOTOX INJECTIONS?

What is BOTOX® Cosmetic?
BOTOX® Cosmetic is a drug that when injected in the region of wrinkles weakens the underlying muscle that causes furrows in the overlying skin. For details, refer to **Chapter 1: What is Botox® and how does it work?**

Am I a candidate for BOTOX® Cosmetic?
Perhaps, the best way to answer that question is to understand what the treatment involves.

The treatment is an office procedure that temporarily smoothes the deep, persistent lines between the brows that develop over time. The treatment involves a few tiny injections that relaxes the muscles that cause those lines to form. No anesthetic is necessary. Some patients opt for ice application just before and after injection. The results generally last 3 to 6 months. Botox® Cosmetic has been widely tested since it was approved by the FDA in April, 2002.

The results are sometimes dramatic, often subtle, and apparent within days. In clinical trials, nearly 90% of the men and women surveyed rated the improvement in the brow lines as moderate to better. For many, Botox® Cosmetic diminishes these lines.

Dr. Mauriello's Commentary: The great advantage of Botox® Cosmetic is that it is fast, simple, and minimally invasive, with no down-time or recovery period. People return directly to work or normal activity following treatment. Once the drug takes effect, patients state that they appear less wrinkled, relaxed, and even refreshed. The results are subtle. The exact change in appearance is difficult even for patient's family or best friend to detect, yet the patient knows that appearance is improved.

BOTOX® Cosmetic is not magical. It will not radically change your appearance nor will it make you look 20 years younger. It will enhance your appearance if you are an appropriate candidate. Botox is injected local into the appropriate muscle so that its effects are targeted for a specific region. It is recommended for all people who wish to improve their tired, wrinkled appearance.

The goal of treatment is not necessarily to look younger but rather to appear refreshed, less harried, and less wrinkled. Answering the following questions may help you decide whether you are a candidate for Botox:

- *Are you concerned about looking and feeling your best?*

- *Do friends, families, and colleagues sometimes say that you appear angry, stressed, or worried or frown without particular reason?*

- *Do you wish to remove lines between the eyebrows so that you would feel better, possibly refreshed and, perhaps, more approachable?*

- *Do you wish to remove forehead lines?*

- *Do you wish to remove the crow's feet in the corner of the eyes?*

- *Do you wish to elevate the eyebrows or one eyebrow?*

- *Do you wish to remove lipstick lines?*

- *Do you wish to have a thicker appearance of the upper and lower lips?*

- *Do you wish to remove horizontal or vertical bands in the neck? Do these bands lie under the skin and are worsened by tensing of the neck muscles?*

- *Do you wish to have any or all of the above changes without losing significant time from work and without having the appearance that you underwent a surgical procedure?*

- *Do you wish to undergo a minimally invasive, relative inexpensive procedure compared to other more involved surgical options, such as facelifts?*

If you answered "yes" to any of these questions, you are probably a candidate for Botox. You must be willing to spend time to see a physician who has significant experience with Botox and who will analyze your facial lines and determine a treatment that is tailored for you. You must then be willing to undergo the treatment as outlined above.

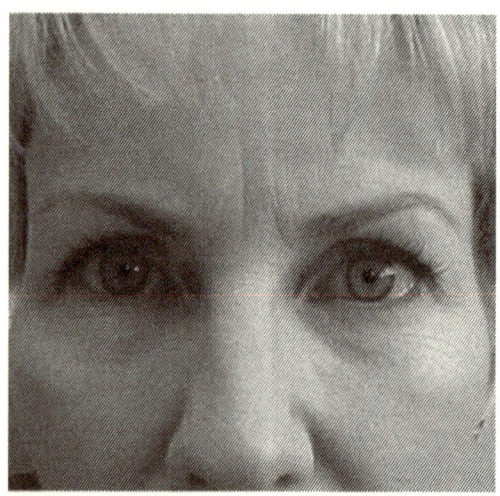

Patient photographed above is a busy executive and has a somewhat harried appearance. She is a candidate for Botox® injections for the frown lines between the eyebrows. (Refer to *CHAPTER 4: WHAT IS THE NATURE OF THE OFFICE EXAMINATION AND BOTOX® TREATMENT OF THE EYEBROW, FOREHEAD, CROW'S FEET, MOUTH, AND NECK REGIONS?* for results after treatment of this actual patient.)

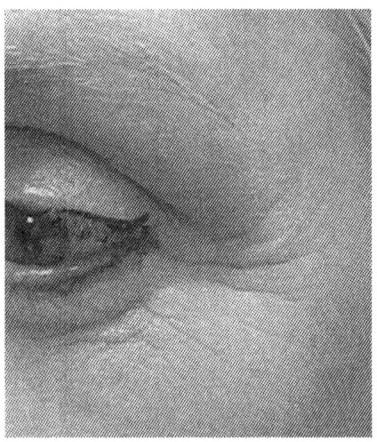

Fine squint lines in the corner of the eyes may be improved with Botox. (Refer to *CHAPTER 4: WHAT IS THE NATURE OF THE OFFICE EXAMINATION AND BOTOX® TREATMENT OF THE EYEBROW, FOREHEAD, CROW'S FEET, MOUTH, AND NECK REGIONS?* for results after treatment of this actual patient.)

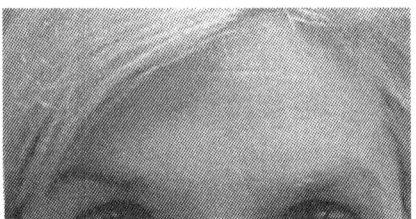

This patient's eyebrows may be elevated and the forehead lines diminished with Botox®. *CHAPTER 4: WHAT IS THE NATURE OF THE OFFICE EXAMINATION AND BOTOX® TREATMENT OF THE EYEBROW, FOREHEAD, CROW'S FEET, MOUTH, AND NECK REGIONS?* for results after treatment of this actual patient.)

Experimental Evidence for Efficacy of Botox

While there is experimental evidence for the efficacy of Botox, Dr. Mauriello's patients can attest to the improvement in their facial wrinkles (See **Chapter 1:** *What is Botox and how does it work?).* This chapter refers to the study funded by Allergan.

FDA has approved the treatment for the frown lines between the eyebrows but the drug has multiple, so-called off label uses. Again, in the experimental studies funded by Allergan Pharmaceuticals, the investigators assessment showed more marked improvement in patients less than 50 years of age or 84.6% as compared to 70.4 in patients ages 50 to 65 years, greater than 50 but less than 65 years and 39.1% in patients over 65 years of age.

The consent form presently used at Dr. Mauriello's office is as follows:

Botulinum Toxin (BOTOX) Consent for Cosmetic Uses

> *As a patient you have the right to be informed about the risks, benefits, and alternatives of any treatment including Botox. Informed consent enhances patient care.*

> *Botulinum toxin injections have been used for more than a decade to improve muscles spasm of the facial muscles. The toxin has been used to correct double vision due to eye muscle disease as well.*

> *Minute amounts of toxin weaken the muscle and improve frown lines, crow's feet in the corner of the eyes and facial expression lines. At this time, Botox has been FDA-approved*

for cosmetic use for brow furrows only at this time. The results with treatment are often quite dramatic but since medicine is not an exact science, no guarantees can be made regarding the results. The results are temporary and more than one treatment session may be necessary to opimize results. Rarely, the drug has no or little effect.

The solution is injected with a small needle. The benefits generally develop over 5 to 14 days.

Side effects and complications have been minimal. Slight swelling and/or bruising may last for several days after injection. Temporary eyelid drooping and brow drooping rarely occur. Infection at the injection site is extremely rare. Rarely, headache, nausea, and flu-like syndrome develop transiently after treatment.

Treatment alternatives, expected benefits, and risks have been explained to me to my satisfaction. As stated in the package insert, "the product contains albumin, a derivative of human blood. Based on effective donor screening and product manufacturing processes, it carries an extremely remote risks for transmission of viral diseases. A theoretical risk for transmission of Cretzfeldt-Jacob disease is extremely rare. No cases of viral disease transmission of Cretzfeldt-Jacob have ever been identified for albumin."

This consent supersedes any previous or written disclosures. I have read and fully understand the above paragraphs and have had sufficient opportunity for open discussion with Dr. Mauriello and to ask questions. I understand Dr. Mauriello has used this drug since 1983 in over 6000 injections (as of

April, 2002) with only minimal, transient side effects in all cases.

I understand that Botox should not be given during pregnancy and that I am not pregnant.

SIGNATURE _____DATE

WITNESS _____DATE

Physician SIGNATURE_____DATE

Dr. Mauriello's commentary: *The consent is somewhat disarming but as with all medical treatment, no result can be guaranteed. The drug is extremely well tolerated in Dr. Mauriello's experience with minimal side-effects.*

Only after an office consultation can the patient determine the possible benefits of Botox injections. The next chapter, **Chapter 3: How do I select a physician to treat me with Botox?**, should be helpful to patients considering Botox® treatment.

CHAPTER 3

HOW DO I SELECT A PHYSICIAN TO TREAT ME WITH BOTOX?

The decision of how to select a physician to inject Botox is somewhat difficult mainly because many different types of physicians perform cosmetic procedures. The consumer, therefore, has a choice and has to exercise good judgment.

Ideally, the consumer should choose a cosmetic surgeon. Cosmetic surgeons may be drawn from the following specialties: dermatology, plastic surgery, maxillofacial surgery (consisting of doctors of dental surgery (DDS) who specialize in the mid-facial area maxilla and the lower face (jaw or mandible), ear nose and throat surgery (otolaryngology) and facial plastic surgery, and finally ophthalmology and oculoplastic surgery (ophthalmic plastic and reconstructive surgery). The latter surgeons specialize in eyelid, both reconstructive and cosmetic, as well tear duct, socket, and orbital surgery. *Ophthalmic plastic and reconstructive (oculoplastic) surgeons) are board-certified in ophthalmology and dedicated to eyelid and other surgeries around the eye.*

What are the backgrounds and training of Ophthalmic Plastic and Reconstructive Surgeons (oculoplastic surgeons)?
The subspecialty of ophthalmic plastic and reconstructive surgery (oculoplastic surgery), is the field of medicine that deals specifically with surgery of the eyelid structures. Most important, because ophthalmic plastic and reconstructive surgeons are board certified ophthalmologists, they have an intimate knowledge of the eye and its supporting structures. Most people are not aware of this subspecialty.

As of 2002, no subspecialty board certifications exist in ophthalmology. Nonetheless, the publish understands that there are retinal specialists, neuro-ophthalmologists, glaucoma experts, and pediatric ophthalmologists. Ophthalmic plastic and reconstructive surgeons are an additional specialty.

The American Society of Ophthalmic Plastic and Reconstructive Surgery (ASOPRS), is the subspecialty society composed of board-certified ophthalmologists who obtain specialized training and credentialing in eyelid, tear duct, socket, and orbital surgery.

ASOPRS Fellows, such as Dr. Mauriello, obtain specialized training after a one-year internship in medicine or surgery and a three to four-year residency in ophthalmology. The ophthalmology residency typically follows four years of college and four years of medical school. This residency includes surgery of the eye and eyelids. As of the year 2000, board-certified (or board-eligible) ophthalmologic surgeons subsequently apply for a two-year fellowship in Ophthalmic Plastic and Reconstructive Surgery approved by the American Society of Ophthalmic

Plastic and Reconstructive Surgery. After completing this training, ASOPRS candidates must pass both an oral and written examination and write a thesis that is approved by the Thesis committee before being inducted into the Society as Fellows. It should be recognized that presently no subspecialty boards exist in any field of ophthalmology. Ophthalmic plastic and reconstructive surgeons are presently attempting to establish a separate Board Certification under the American Board of Ophthalmology.

Ophthalmologists are most familiar with BOTOX since botulinum toxin type A was developed by an ophthalmologist, Dr. Alan Scott, a Pacific Medical Center, to straighten eyes with improper alignment in the late 1970's. The drug was later used by ophthalmologists to treat involuntary eyelid spasms. Presently, this drug is used by cosmetic surgeons in all disciplines to improve wrinkles in the face.

Should I go to a surgeon who advertises ?
Increasingly, doctors are advertising their talents. Some surgeons hire a publicist at great expense in order to obtain "brand name" recognition. Such physicians are often quoted in woman's magazines and may, in fact, provide free surgical care to writers and editors of the magazines. These surgeons may incur great expense and ultimately, if they are successful, have a high volume practice. Volume is not a guarantee of quality although practice does tend to improve surgical results. The media have reported that some surgeons may perform surgery on radio station and television personalities as well as magazine editors, in order to win their favor and acclaim.

The best referral is from another patient who has obtained treatment. Nonetheless, advertising provides the individual doctor with a forum to make his credentials, training, and expertise known to the public. For these reasons, advertising will probably increase in the future. Certainly, a patient should not be dissuaded from arranging a consultation with a surgeon who advertises.

The thrust of Dr. Mauriello's advertising is educational and therefore attempts to inform the public of the training and experience of ophthalmic plastic and reconstructive surgeons.

What is the best way to find an ophthalmic plastic and reconstructive surgeon?
The best way to find a surgeon is to contact the American Society of Ophthalmic Plastic and Reconstructive Surgery in Winter Park, Florida (**www.asoprs.org**).

Are only ophthalmic plastic and reconstructive (oculoplastic) surgeons capable of performing and advancing the field of cosmetic eyelid surgery?
As Dr. Mauriello stated in his text, *Beautiful Eyes Consumer guide to cosmetic eyelid surgery,* Dr. Mauriello agrees with Robert Goldwyn, MD, a plastic surgeon and Editor-in-Chief of Plastic and Reconstructive Surgery Journal. At the 28th Annual Scientific Symposium of the ASOPRS on October 25th, 1997 in San Francisco, Dr. Goldwyn stated that surgical procedures should be performed by any surgeon who is able to benefit the patient regardless of background.

Surgeons of all disciplines should avoid a cookie cutter approach to cosmetic surgery and determine what, in fact, is bothering the patient. Ideally, the patient should ask the surgeon what complications may occur during the course of your surgery. Ophthalmic plastic and reconstructive (oculoplastic) surgeons have training in ophthalmology and are able to handle virtually all complications.

What questions should I ask in the consultation in order to determine whether the physician should treat me?
Each patient should decide on a physician based on the credentials and background of the physician. In addition, the patient should determine the frequency that the physician has performed a given procedure. The patient must be comfortable with the informed consent provided by the treating doctor as well as the recommendations of other physicians and friends who have undergone Botox treatment.

However, only after a personal consultation is the individual patient able to best select a physician to perform their Botox treatment. The only way to make a final decision is to meet the doctor and ask him to show photographs of actual patient results. Frankly, no physician is able to comment directly on another physician's abilities unless the first physician has operated with that physician and personally observed that surgeon's results over time. Indeed, it is rare for surgeons to be able to truly judge the work of fellow surgeons.

The average person does not have the time to do exhaustive research on any given surgeon. It is reasonable to ask the physician how many specific procedures the physician performs per week. A phone conversation with the last few patients that the physician has treated may be worthwhile.

Many times, the patient must rely on the judgment and the positive chemistry between the patient and the treating physician.

CHAPTER 4

WHAT IS THE NATURE OF THE OFFICE EXAMINATION AND BOTOX® TREATMENT OF THE EYEBROW, FOREHEAD, CROW'S FEET, MOUTH, AND NECK REGIONS

What muscles will the doctor weaken to remove facial lines?
Wrinkles or rhytides are exaggerated by forceful contracture of muscles as occurs after forced closure of the eyelids. Skin changes including loss of elasticity and ground substance in the dermis also cause wrinkles. These changes are discussed in *Chapter 5—How do I take care of my skin to prevent wrinkles?*

The muscle activity causing wrinkles is evident in the photographs below. *Botox works by selective temporary weakening of specific muscles.* Knowledge of the anatomy is critical to the physician's successful use of Botox. Minimal doses of Botox® are optimally used in order to avoid weakening other nearby muscles that are not the target muscles that need to be treated to reduce the wrinkles.

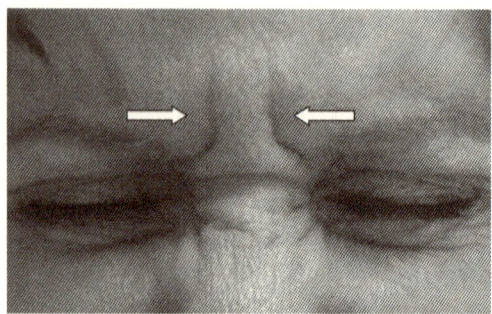

In the above photograph, note the contraction of the eyebrow muscles, known as the corrugator muscle and another muscle, the depressor supracilii, causes vertically oriented lines as shown in the patient photographed above. The horizontal white arrows demonstrate how the brows come together due to contraction of these muscles. The depressor supracilii muscle is part of the orbicularis oculi muscle that surrounds the eye and closes the eyelids.

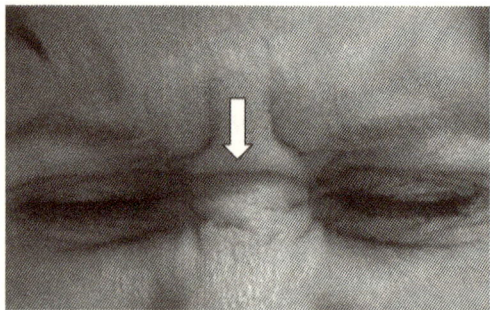

Horizontal lines in the skin of the nose are mainly due to contraction of the muscle known as the procerus muscle. This muscle is superficial and lies just beneath the skin. The corrugator and depressor supracilii muscles are located underneath this muscle. The vertical white arrow indicates the direction of contracture of the procerus muscle.

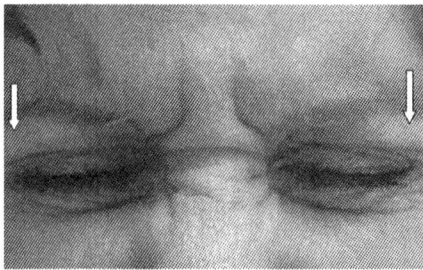

The muscle known as the orbicularis muscle lowers the outer parts of the brow. The orbicularis muscle surrounds the eye and closes the eye by lowering the upper lid and raising the lower lid. In addition, its effect on the brow is indicated by the vertical white arrows in the photograph above. The procerus muscle, the corrugator muscles, and the the orbicularis oculi muscle contract and thereby lower the nasal portion of the brow. These contractions cause frowning.

The frowning muscles help lower the brow, and also decrease the distance between the nasal portions of the brow.

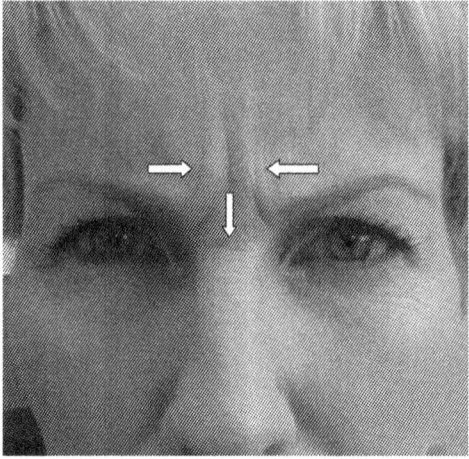

In the patient photographed above, the muscles that cause frowning lower the brow and decrease the distance between the nasal portions of the brow. In the patient photographed above, the effect of the procerus muscle contraction is indicated by the vertical white arrow and corrugator and depressor supercilii by the horizontal white arrows.

The orbicularis oculi muscle is a superficial, circular muscle that encompasses the upper and lower lid and surrounds the eye. It closes the eyelid and pulls the brow down. The depressor supracilii is one of the muscles in the nasal group of muscles that along with the orbicularis oculi muscle, helps bring the nasal part of the brow downward.

Weakening of all the muscles (the corrugator and procerus muscles and the upper lid orbicularis oculi muscle) depicted in the photograph above elevates the eyebrow. The weakening occurs selectively in the same vertical plane that the particular muscle is weakened. Botox® works by selectively weakening these muscles.

The space between the eyebrows is widened after Botox. In order to decrease the forehead lines, the frontalis muscle, a brow elevator is weakened. Weakening the frontalis muscle may cause eyebrow drooping. Therefore, injections in anatomic sites adjacent to the frontalis muscle must be given discretely in order to avoid lowering the eyebrow.

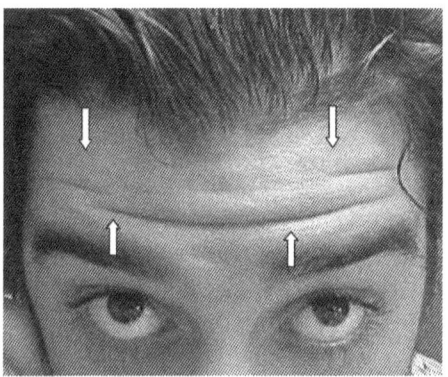

The vertical arrows in the photograph above show the direction of the contraction of the frontalis muscle that elevates the eyebrow. The frontalis muscle elevates the eyebrow and lowers the hairline. The effect is to decrease the distance between the eyebrows and the scalp. The frontalis muscle is vertically oriented and the arrows show its activity. Selective weakening of the frontalis muscle with Botox ® may lower the entire eyebrow.

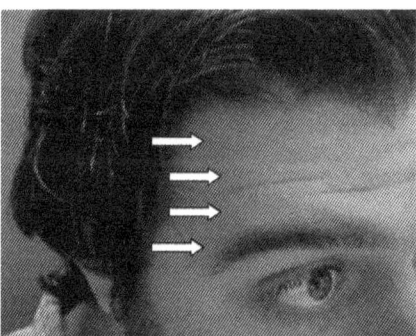

In the photograph above, the tips of the white arrows show the end of the frontalis muscle that elevates the eyebrow. The frontalis muscle extends across the forehead, but the muscle usually does not extend beyond the eyebrow (towards the ear). Its extent is variable in every individual. Arrows indicate the outer margin of frontalis muscle. Its outer margin inserts in the bone of the forehead. This line may be felt as a ridge of bone on your own forehead. The outer border of the frontalis muscle is evident when the patient bites down and the masseter muscle that contributes to chewing (mastication) is felt just outside the frontalis muscle's outer border. The orbicularis oculi muscle circles around the eyes and is present just under the skin. The muscle fibers in the upper eyelid pull the eyebrow down. Your physician may weaken the orbicularis muscle without weakening the elevation of the eyebrow. He treats the outer aspect of the upper eyelid since the frontalis muscle is not present in that location and the risk of causing the eyebrow to droop is unlikely.

The best way to determine whether you are a candidate for Botox injections is to obtain a consultation and speak to an expert to consider treatment of specific areas of the face. The most popular area of treatment is between the brows.

Treatment of vertical and oblique frown lines with Botox®
Wrinkles are improved by Botox. The effects generally last 3 to 6 months.

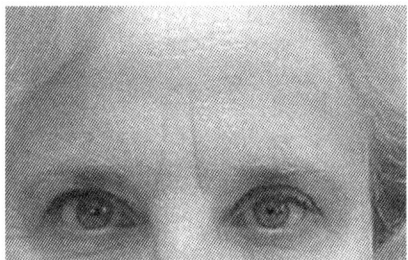
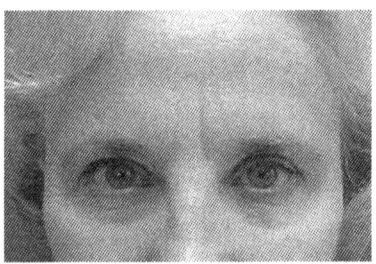

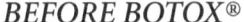

BEFORE BOTOX®   *AFTER BOTOX®*

Before treatment (top left) and after treatment (top, right), the space between the eyebrows is widened and the vertical lines softened as compared to before treatment . Overall, the entire face appears more open after treatment. The patient did not wish any other areas treated.

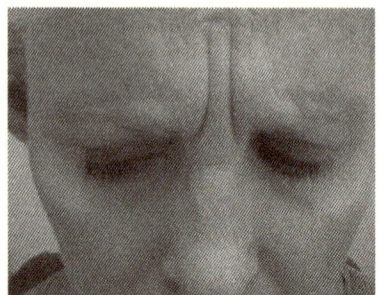 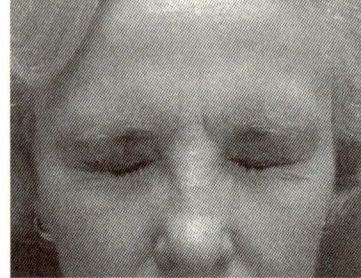

BEFORE BOTOX®   *TWO WEEKS AFTER BOTOX®*

The intensity of the muscle contraction after treatment (top, right) is diminished as compared to forced contraction before treatment (top, left). The intensity of voluntary forced contracture is significantly decreased intensity 2 weeks after Botox injection.

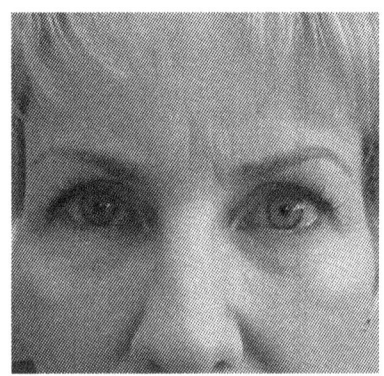
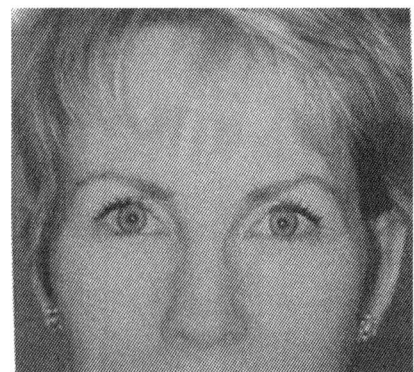

BEFORE BOTOX®   *AFTER BOTOX®*

Frown lines (top, right) are improved after Botox (top, left). Space between the eyebrows is increased after treatment and patient has a less harried appearance.

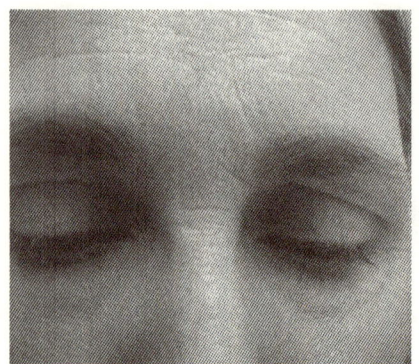 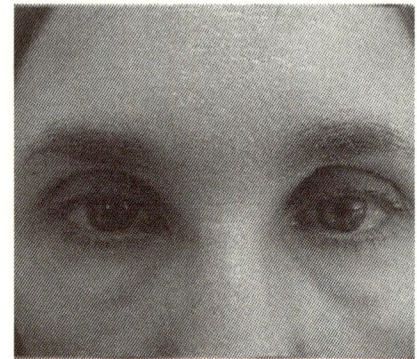

BEFORE BOTOX®   **_AFTER BOTOX®_**

Forehead lines and frown lines (top,left) temporarily minimized by Botox (top, right).

Elevation of the eyebrow with Botox

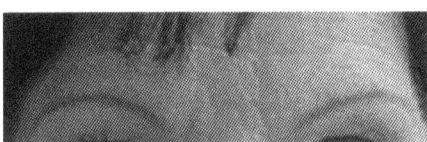 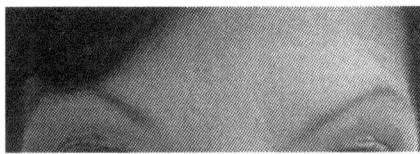

BEFORE BOTOX®   *AFTER BOTOX®*

Before treatment (top left), the wrinkles above the brow and forehead are evident.

Widening of space between the eyebrows and the softening of vertical lines between eyebrows (top, right) is apparent after treatment. The eyebrows also appear elevated in their outer aspect after treatment. (Parts of photographs are obscured to maintain patient's confidentiality).

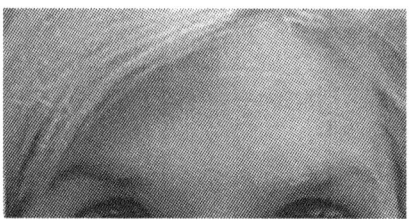

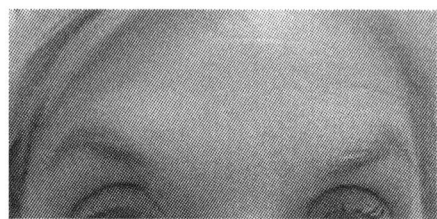

BEFORE BOTOX®   *AFTER BOTOX®*

Elevation of entire brow and the widening of distance between the eyebrows is evident after Botox® treatment (top, right), as compared to the appearance prior to treatment (top, right). The entire forehead is vertically lengthened. There is also softening of the lines in the brow area and forehead after Botox ® treatment (Part of photograph is obscured to maintain patient's confidentiality).

Elevation of upper eyelid with Botox

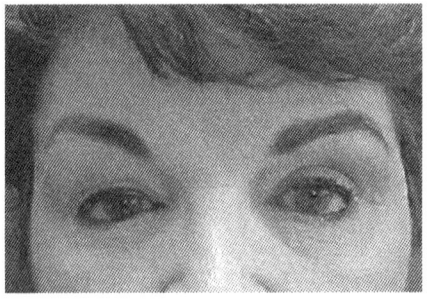 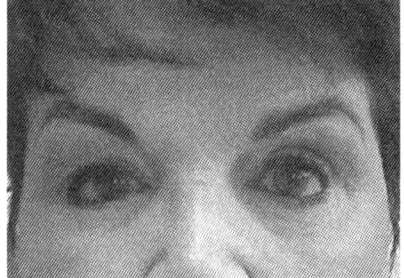

BEFORE BOTOX®   *AFTER BOTOX®*

The right upper lid is slightly lower than the left upper eyelid before Botox treatment (top, left). After Botox injection (top, right), the right brow is more elevated and arched and the frown lines appear softer. In addition, the right upper eyelid is elevated.

Should I have an eyebrow lift?
Many surgeons presently favor procedures that surgically elevate the eyebrows. Such procedures may be performed with small incisions in the scalp and facilitated by the use of endoscopes. However, it should be kept in mind that the Eyebrows basically frame the entire face as well as the eyelids. Any change in contour and elevation of the eyebrows may change one's facial appearance. Eyebrow lifts, in Dr. Mauriello's opinion, are important when the brows are not at the same level.

Office Botox may be used to simulate an eyelid lift. The effects are temporary. Yet, any given patient may determine whether surgical correction is necessary after undergoing Botox treatment:

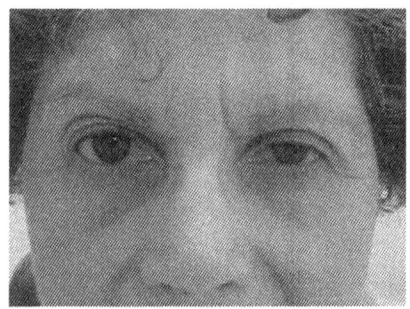 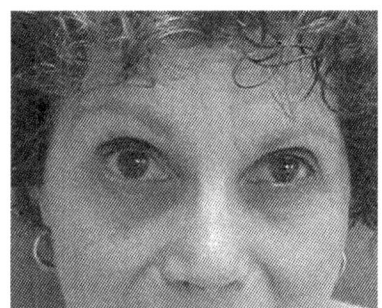

BEFORE BOTOX®   *AFTER BOTOX®*

The right upper lid is slightly lower than left upper eyelid before Botox treatment (top, left). After Botox injection (top, right), the left brow is only slightly more elevated, but there is softening of the frown lines and widening of the space between the eyebrows. The left upper eyelid is elevated after treatment.

Treatment of horizontal lines above eyebrow with Botox ®

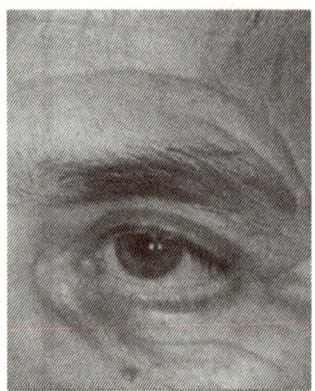 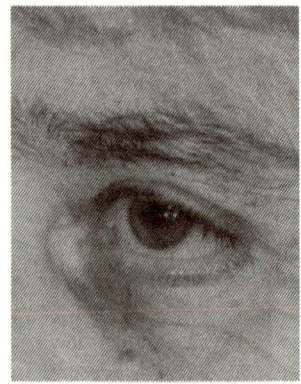

BEFORE BOTOX®   *AFTER BOTOX®*

This patient underwent treatment of lines above eyebrow (top, left). Note effect of Botox (top, right) after treatment just above the outer aspect of the brow.

Treatment of crow's feet (squint) lines with Botox®

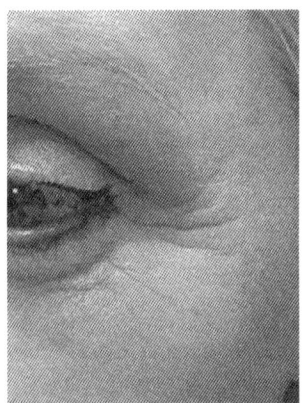 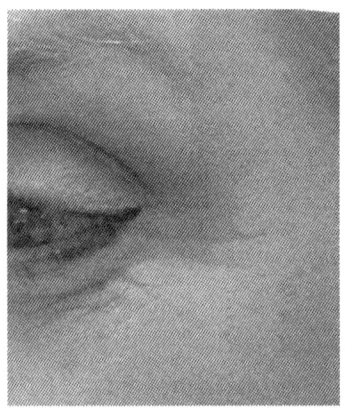

BEFORE BOTOX®   **AFTER BOTOX®**

Crow's feet (winkles lines in the corners on the eyes) may also be treated with Botox. Subtle improvement may be seen in crow's feet after Botox treatment (top, right). Patient is not smiling. Lower facial lines were not treated to avoid loss of facial expression.

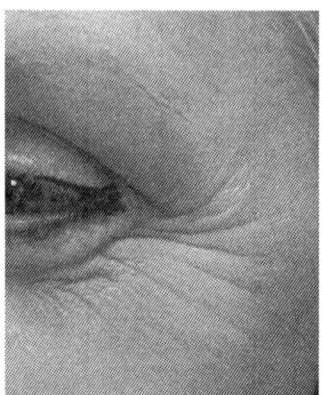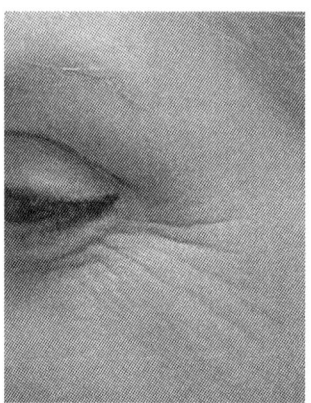

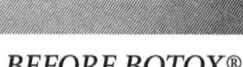**BEFORE BOTOX®**   **AFTER BOTOX®**

Crow's feet (winkles lines in the corners on the eyes) are shown before treatment when smiling ((top, right) and after Botox treatment (top, right). There is still evidence of facial animation yet the lines in the corner of the eyes are diminished. Lower facial lines were not treated and patient is, therefore, still able to smile.

Treatment of lipstick lines and thickening with eversion of lips with Botox ®

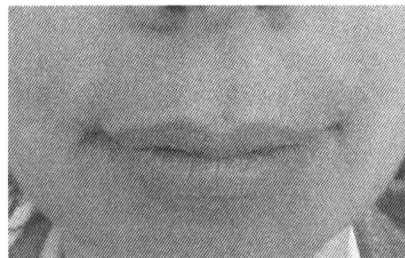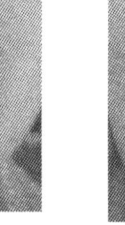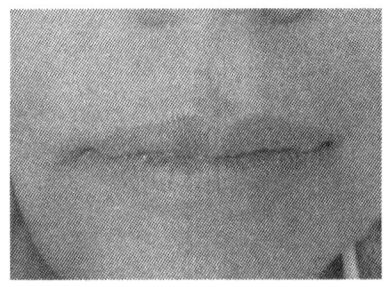

BEFORE BOTOX®   *AFTER BOTOX®*

Note thickening of lips and slight eversion after Botox treatment of lips on each side of Cupid's bow.

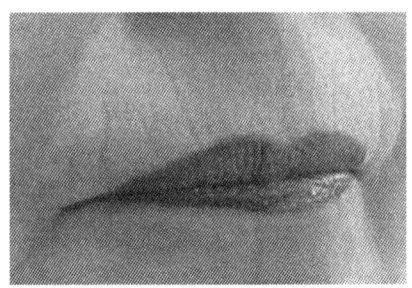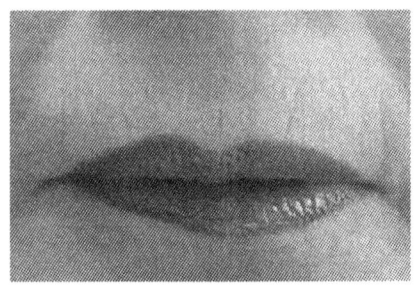

BEFORE BOTOX®   *AFTER BOTOX®*

Lipstick lines (top, left) are diminished by Botox (top, right)

Treatment of neck bands with Botox®

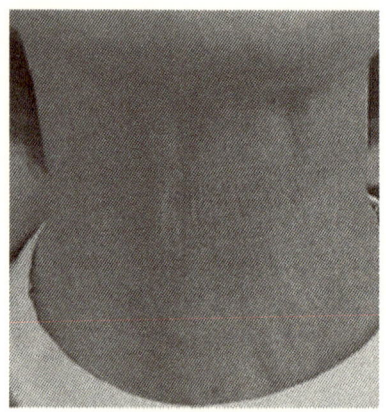 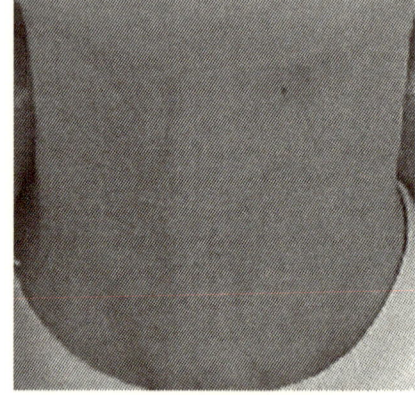

BEFORE BOTOX®   *AFTER BOTOX®*

Vertical platysmal band on the patients right side (left) is greatly reduced in its severity after treatment with Botox (right).

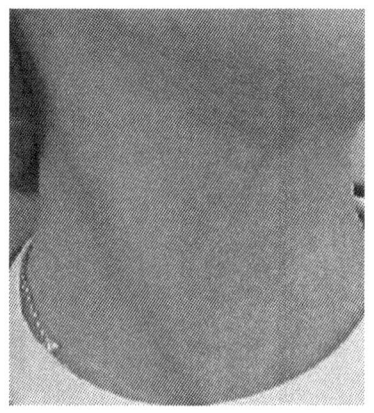
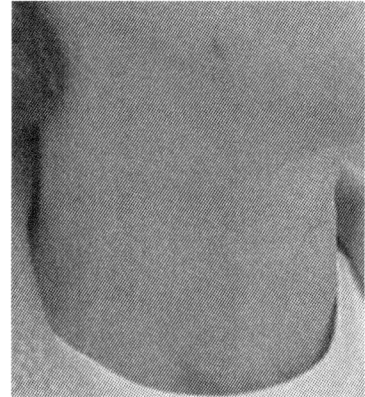

BEFORE BOTOX®   *AFTER BOTOX®*

It is important to recognize that although the effects are temporary, over time, there appears to be a definite cumulative and
possibly a long-lasting effect.

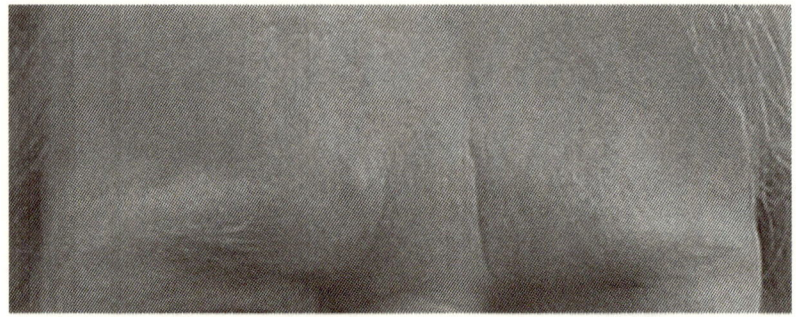

In photograph above, vertical lines are evident between eyebrows prior to first treatment with Botox ®.

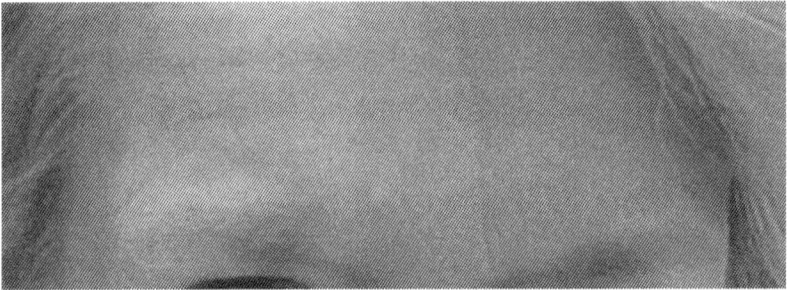

Prior to fourth treatment, vertical lines between eyebrows are much less evident than before any treatment was started in above photograph.

How is the treatment performed?
Your doctor will analyze your concerns and your particular facial musculature, and then treat those areas that may be improved. Photographic documentation of the eyelids and facial muscle, both with and without animation, are critical before and after treatment.

The procedure is performed in the office. After cleansing the skin, minute amounts of the reconstituted Botox ® are injected with a very small gauge needle. Generally, no anesthetic is necessary. Sometimes patients opt for ice application before and after the injections. The discomfort does not continue after the Botox ® is injected.

Dr. Mauriello's technique is to use the lowest dose to accomplish the purpose and thereby minimize complications. He sees patients at two-week intervals initially when they are first treated in order to determine the effect of minimal doses on specific muscle groups.

Once the appropriate muscle groups that are to be treated are determined along with the optimum dose, the injections are repeated at one treatment session. Injections are deferred for at least 4 months. There appears to be a cumulative effect of injections.

How do I help eliminate the nasolabial lines?
Botox treatment is not good for the often deep lines that extend from the outer corners of the nostrils to the outer corners of the mouth. This lines are known as the nasolabial folds. These are

best treated presently with fillers such as collagen or hyaluronic acid (soon to be FDA-approved).

Hyaluronic acid—the new dynamic filler to replace collagen?
A new treatment involves a drug known as Restylane. This drug is planned to be approved by the FDA in early 2003. It is already available in Canada.

Restylane is a synthetic compound, hyaluronic acid, that is a naturally occurring chemical known as a glycosaminoglycan (GAG). GAG is a vital component of all connective tissues. Hyaluronic acid may be thought of as the glue that holds the collagen in place. GAG's have water-binding capacities that enhance the effect of this filler material and correct wrinkles and skin foldings. GAG's decrease with age and benefit from replenishment. Presently this material is injected into the joints of patients with osteoporosis. Hyaluronic acid is the material the fills the back of the eye, the vitreous.

Hyaluronic acid injections serve to replenish the loss of this matrix materially that occurs with aging. Hyaluronic acid is naturally occurring in rooster combs, bacterial cultures, umbilical cord, vitreous of the eye, tendons, and skin.

Unlike collagen, no need for skin testing with Restylane: Since hyaluronic acid has a uniform chemical structure throughout nature, there are no potential for immunologic reactions to Restylane. Collagen or bovine origin, in contrast, requires skin testing in the doctor's office to determine whether an individual is sensitive. The patient must wait 4 weeks after testing to determine whether there is a reaction. This testing is not necessary with Restylane. Hyaluronic acid is degraded very quickly within 1 to 2 days by the body's enzymes and then is converted to carbon dioxide and water in the liver.

Restylane is produced in various concentrations that have specific uses to reduce wrinkles:

Restylane Fine Lines—at 20 mg/ml concentration, contains 200 gel particles per ml is used to treat fine superficial lines (For superficial dermis)

Restylane—100-gel particles per milliliter is designed to treat deeper wrinkles such as eyebrow folds, deep lines that extend from the outer corners of the nostrils to the outer corners of the mouth (nasolabial lines) and is also used as a lip filler (For the mid-dermis)

Perlane— 8-gel particles per ml is employed to treat the junction of lower dermis and subcutis as well as the deep folds in the nasolabial area. It is also used as a lip filler

Perlane Plus—4-gel particles per ml (most viscous or thickest form)

Restylane appears to lasts for 8 to 12 months as compared to collagen that last 3 to 6 months.

The material requires administration with a fine needle into the wrinkles in the skin.

COSMETIC EYELID SURGERY REJUVENATES THE ENTIRE FACE

While facial cosmetic Botox provide relief without the permanent effects of surgery, the rejuvenating effects of eyelid surgery without any Botox treatment are shown below:

4-LID COSMETIC EYELID SURGERY

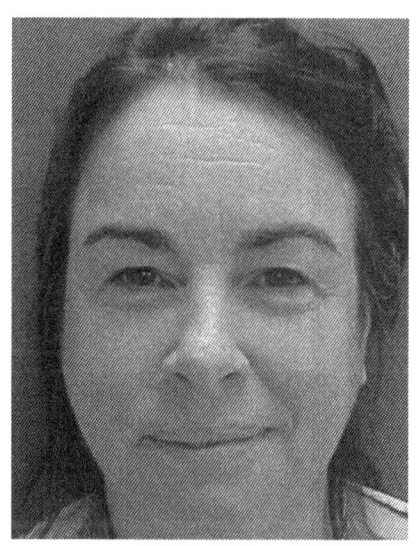 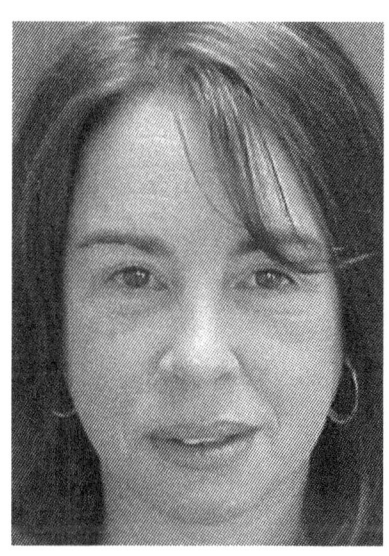

BEFORE SURGERY   *2 WEEKS AFTER SURGERY*

This patient no the way photographed below received Botox treatment.

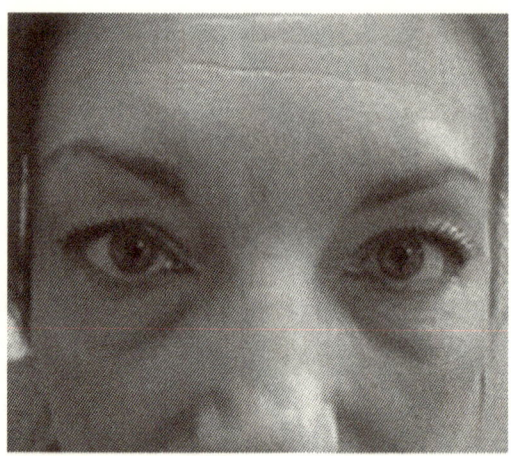

BEFORE

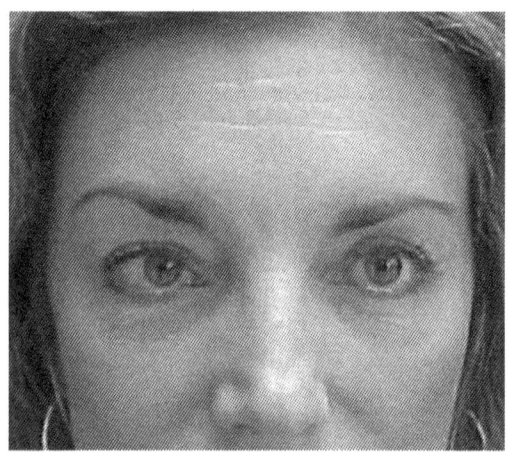

4 MONTHS AFTER SURGERY
Note elevation of cheek.

Dr. Mauriello considered the entire subject of cosmetic eyelid surgery in **Beautiful Eyes: Consumer guide to cosmetic eyelid surgery.** This book is available on the web at amazon.com.

CHAPTER 5

HOW DO I TAKE CARE OF MY SKIN TO PREVENT WRINKLES?

Importance of Skin Care

Skin care helps to protect the skin against photoaging (aging due to sun exposure) and skin cancer. Skin care products thicken the skin and improve uneven pigmentation of the skin. Ultimately, skin care enhances the beneficial effects of Botox injections, eyelid surgery, or any facial surgery. Skin care alone rejuvenates. Skin care may be improved by home care regimens that do not have the risks of deeper chemical peels or laser resurfacing. Skin care at home requires a commitment of time and does involve expense. Nonetheless, the results are gratifying especially when performed under the supervision of a physician who is dedicated to skin care. This section considers over -the-counter, as well as prescription, medications. A background discussion of the anatomy of the skin is helpful. (This section has been updated and extracted in part from **Beautiful Eyes: Consumer Guide to Cosmetic Eyelid Surgery.**)

Dr. Mauriello's Commentary: It is important to maintain the effect of the cosmetic eyelid surgery and to enhance the effects of Botox®. Ask your surgeon about skin care. Such care is also important to help prevent skin cancers.

LAYERS OF SKIN:
> *Epidermis—has superficial keratin, a horny protective layer*
> *Dermis—contains collagen, elastic tissue and ground substance*
>> *papillary dermis—superficial*
>> *reticular dermis—deep*
> *subcutaneous tissue*

The outermost layer of skin or epidermis is composed of epithelial cells, known as **keratinocytes,** that have a protective role. The most superficial part of the epidermis is the *stratum corneum* or horny layer produced by the underlying cells of the epidermis and composed of keratin. The keratin in the stratum corneum protects against physical damage but also, to some extent, against sun exposure. It is most developed on the palms of the hands and the soles of the feet in order to protect these areas from the minor traumas of daily living.

Melanin, the brown skin pigment, is present in the epidermis and, like melanin throughout the body, it is produced by specialized cells known as melanocytes. The melanin protects the skin surface against ultraviolet light by absorbing it. For this reason, skin cancers are extremely rare in black persons and darkly pigmented races.

Hair follicles are associated with sebaceous glands that express their sebum or oil into the lumen of the hair follicle to serve as an inherent cooling system and as lubrication of the overlying skin. The great number of pilosebaceous units distinguish facial skin from skin elsewhere in the body. The nose and forehead have more sebaceous units than the cheeks or temples.

With age, the hairs turn gray due to decreased production of melanin by melanocytes in the bulbs of the hair follicle.

Photoaging (aging due to sun exposure)

So-called **photoaging** of the skin results from ultraviolet (UV) light exposure and is cumulative over years. Sun damage results in the following changes in the skin:

- wrinkles
- dark blotches
- freckles
- leathery texture
- loss of elasticity

In addition, the skin is predisposed to skin cancers such as basal cell carcinoma, squamous cell carcinoma, and melanoma. Sun blocks are absolutely essential in preventing these cancers and should be used by everyone.

Microscopic view of photoaging or sun-damaged skin

Aged, sun-damaged skin causes the superficial epidermis of the skin to lose its translucency and to appear dry, rough, and dull skin. So-called benign keratosis develop. In addition, ephelides (freckles) are noted in increased numbers due to accumulation of granules of the brown pigment (melanin) in the lower layer of cells of the epidermis, known as the basal and suprabasal keratinocytes. The keratinocytes are the cells that constitute the epidermis.

Breakdown of elastic tissue in the dermis of the skin occurs with sun exposure and age
With age and sun damage, the normal elastic tissue in the dermis of the skin breaks down. Macrophages are specialized cells that repair damage and degeneration throughout the tissues of the body. These cells engulf the broken down coarse granules. The elastotic breakdown material accumulates and crowds out the normal collagenous fibers that are also degenerating and resorbing with age. The normal collagen fibers provide the framework of the skin. The elastotic material is resorbed and, ultimately, the total volume of the dermis diminishes. Since there is relatively too much epidermis for the shrinking dermis, wrinkles appear on the skin surface.

Increase in pigment production by specialized pigment cells, melanocytes: Another type of cell, the melanocyte, produces the skin pigment, melanin. Melanocytes increase in number in the lower or basal layer of epidermis and result in solar lentigos (liver spot) in which the amount of melanin or brown pigment increases in each melanocyte and also in the basal keratinocytes (cells of the epidermis at its lowest portion). Specialized macrophages, known as dermal melanophages, migrate into in the dermis with the sole purpose of imbibing and digesting dispersed melanin pigment. In addition, comedones that plug the openings of pilosebaceous units develop with photoaging or sun damage.

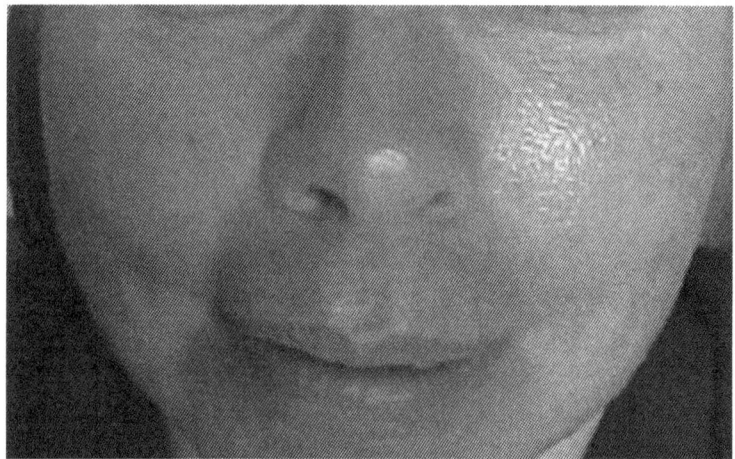

Pigmentary changes around the mouth tend to worsen in summer months due to sun exposure as shown in above photograph.

> **Decrease in tissue matrix of dermis:** *The ground substance or matrix of the dermis contains glycosaminoglycans (GAG's) that have excellent water binding capacity and serve to hydrate the skin. The GAG's decrease with age and add to the shrinkage of the dermis. Restylane injections help replenish this deficit (see the end of* **Chapter 4: Office examination and treatment of eyebrow, forehead, crow's feet, mouth, and neck regions**

Treatment of sun-damaged skin

SUN BLOCK: An effective sun block is the basis of all skin care. Excess ultraviolet B (UVB) rays occur in 290-320nm cause skin burns while UVAII short rays (320-340nm) and UVAI long rays (340-400nm) are responsible for photoaging. These latter rays may lead to skin cancer.

Zine oxide is a sun block. A sun block creates a *physical* block to the sun rays. A sun block is not absorbed by thebody and provides broad spectrum protection against UVA/UVB. from 290 nm to 380 nm.

Sun screen: In contrast to a sun block, a sun screen is absorbed by the superficial epidermis and metabolized or broken down by the body to potentially cause allergy.
The most common chemical sun screen, octyl methoxycinnamate (OMC), is absorbed by the epidermis of the skin. It only blocks the UVB. burning rays, not the long UVA rays that cause photoaging.

In summary, sun blocks and sun screens, to be equivalent , must inhibit the damaging effects of the broad spectrum of ultraviolet light. It is, therefore, important to select with your physician one that has a broad effect against the UVA and UVB rays. In addition, the sun block is not absorbed by the epidermis of the skin and, therefore, allergy to sun block is less likely to develop than with a sun screen.

Antioxidants: In addition to sun screens and sun blocks, antioxidants protect against photoaging by neutralizing reactive oxygen species or free radicals that damage skin at the cellular level. A free radical is an atom or group of atoms with at least one unpaired electron. Each unpaired electron looks for another electron with which to bond and chemical reactions occur until each unpaired electron has a mate. Sun (UV) exposure, smoking, and pollution depletes antioxidants.

Antioxidants—Vitamin C and E, zinc, alpha lipoic acid, and dihydrolipolate, glutathione

Topical vitamin-C (L-Ascorbic acid form) is a powerful antioxidant that in the laboratory enhances collagen (fibrous tissue formation) synthesis. Collagen thickens the dermis of skin and, thereby, decreases wrinkles. Vitamin C products, in general, improve skin tone, elasticity and firmness of skin by collagen synthesis and prevent photoaging by their antioxidant effect. Aging skin, as previously discussed, is characterized by loss of collagen.

Vitamin C derivatives, such as ascorbyl palmitate and magnesium ascorbyl phosphate, commonly found in many skin care products and listed as ingredients on the products' labels. These products may not be absorbed or converted to the active L-ascorbic acid form in high enough concentrations to have an antioxidant effect. It is important that vitamin C is pure, bioavailable (the active vitamin C penetrates the skin), and stable. Concentrations for the eyelids are lower (5%) than in the facial area (10-20%) in order to avoid skin irritation and redness. The eyelid creams or gels smooth the puffy appearance of eyelids.

These vitamin C treatments are expensive to produce. It is advisable to select one with your physician that is effective. *Many inexpensive, over-the-counter products may not be beneficial.* The vitamin C products tend not to be stable and, therefore, it is necessary to determine the shelf-life of any such cream purchased.

Vitamin E is dependent on vitamin C because the latter vitamin helps regenerate vitamin E. Both vitamin C and E prevent suppression of immunity induced by sun exposure (UV light), have anti-inflammatory effects, and promote healing. Alpha lipoic acid regenerates vitamin C. Only vitamin E (alpha tocopheral) is the stable, active form. Vitamin E esters (acetate, succinate linoleate, nicotinate) found in many cosmetic foundations are not antioxidants.

Zinc works similarly to vitamin C but does not help regenerate vitamin. E. However, zinc helps the body maintain proper levels blood levels of Vitamin E. Zinc stabilizes lipid or cell membranes. Also, zinc and bioflavonoids firm and smooth skin.

> *Dr. Mauriello's Commentary: It is important that products containing high concentrations of antioxidants, are stable, and bioavailable (biologically active at the site applied).*

Retinoids or tretinoins (Retin-A): Retinoids are a great advance in skin care and require a prescription. Their effects are quite dramatic when they are used assiduously and judiciously as prescribed by a physician.

Retin-A (Ortho Pharmaceutical Corporation, Raritan, NJ) has the following effects:

- helps decrease hyperpigmentation (dark pigmentation) and, therefore, it may be helpful after a chemical peel (or laser resurfacing)
- increases collagen formation (new fibrous tissue formation)

- promotes healing which is useful after any injury such as chemical peels, laser resurfacing, and dermabrasion
- promotes new blood vessel formation associated with healing (angiogenesis) which may lead to prolonged skin erythema (redness)

Renova (Ortho Pharmaceutical Corporation) containing tretinoin 0.05% in a water may diminish irritant dermatosis that may occur with Retin-A.

Tretinoins cause skin redness and flakiness: The main problem with tretinoins is the irritation they induce. Redness (erty-hema), flakiness, and increased skin sensitivity persist 2 -4 weeks after treatment. This irritation often does subside if treatment is continued. There may be a true allergy to butylated hydroxytoluene, a preservative used. In this case, your physician will recommend that the product be discontinued.

Use tretinoins at night: A light sensitivity (photosensitivity) may result from thinning of the stratum corneum. Sunlight may breakdown tretinoin and, therefore, tretinoin should be used at night. Tretinoin induced photosensitivity may be exacerbated by thiazides, tetracyclines, phenothiazines, fluroquinolones and sulfonamides.

The preparation should be chosen which is least irritating and should be started with lowest concentration. Tretinoin is available as follows (the cream is more moisturizing):

Retin-A cream	0.025
	0.05%
	0.1%

Retin-A gel	0.01%
	0.025%
Retin-A solution	0.05%
Renova (water in light mineral oil emulsion)*	0.05%
Retina-A Microcream**	0.1%

Renova may be less irritating as may Retin-A Microcream. The latter forms microscopic porous beads without the use of oils or organic solvents like ethanol or acetone that may cause skin drying and irritation. A third generation tretinoin, Differin 0.1% gel (Galderma, Fort Worth, Texas), possibly produces less irritation and no phototoxicity. In addition, tretinoins may aggravate acne rosacea and atopic dermatitis as well as acne vulgaris (common acne).

Tretitoins should be applied to a clean well-dried face at night. They should be started on an every other night basis or every third night on patients with extremely sensitive skin. Gradually, the tretinoins are increased to nightly use. Tretinoins may be drying.

In patients with sensitive skin, particularly during the summer, tretinoins may be started every third night. All abrasive soaps, cleansers, and scrubs should be discontinued. Any high concentration of alcohol and astringents with their drying effect should be scrupulously avoided.

Wait 30 minutes before applying a moisturizer after tretinoin.

Other over-the-counter skin care products: **In addition to sun blocks and screens, and the tretinoins, other products are helpful and are listed below.**

Aloe, rosemary, cucumber, and green tea are calming botanical extracts which also have anti-inflammatory effects and help soothe, lighten, and refresh tired, sagging skin.

Chamomile has a soothing and calming, emollient or soothing and softening effect.

Thyme extract also helps to soothe skin by increasing blood circulation. It may help soften but not eliminate the dark circles under the eye. There are no controlled studies to demonstrate the efficacy of these products although many such products are touted commercially.

In contrast, **alpha hydroxy acids (glycolic and lactic acid)** have a long track record of exfoliating rough, textured outer layer of skin to smoothing the skin.

Other common alpha-hydroxy carbolic acids—
        mandolic acid
        malic acid
        tartaric acid
        citric acid
        pyruvic acid
        benzylic acid
        tropic acid

kojic acid lightens skin by inhibiting production of melanin

Alpha-hydroxy acids (AHAs)—thicken epidermis, collagen in papillary dermis, and ground substance in dermis: AHA's help to thicken the skin by thickening the surface epidermis and the papillary dermis (superficial dermis) with new collagen and acid mucopolysaccharide, the material in dermis' ground substance. The quality of elastic fibers improves as does the even distribution of brown melanin. AHA's also cause diminished abnormal keratinization of the surface epidermis. There may be less irritation than with tretinoins.

Combining AHA's with tretinoins may not cause any greater irritation than with tretinoins alone and may improve dyspigmentation (abnormal skin pigmentation) more than with the use of tretinoin alone. Glycolic acids range from 40 to 70% and may be applied at weekly or biweekly intervals. The higher concentrations of AHA's are sometimes used by physicians as chemical peels, but they tend to have a drying effect.

AHA's may be applied in the morning to a clean face.

Hydroquinones—prevent new melanin (brown pigment) formation: Hydroquinone does not bleach out existing pigment but does prevent the production of new brown melanin pigment in the skin. The drug inhibits tyrosinase, the enzyme that enables melanocytes in the skin to produce melanin, the brown skin pigment. Pigment irregularities with no visible changes in the skin usually result from sun exposure and are exacerbated by any hormonal change such as pregnancy, oral contraceptive use, and menopause.

Irritation may result from hydroquinones and the concentration may be decreased. The concentrations range from 4% up to 8%. A solution or gel may be more irritating than a moisturizing cream base. In some patients, a hydrocortisone to decrease inflammation may be necessary. Patients with an unusual condition, known as oochronosis, may develop permanent brown discoloration within the dermis after use of hydroquinone. Hydroquinone should not be used in any patient with this rare condition.

The solution, gel, or cream formulation is used in the morning or twice daily. It may be combined as a 4 to 8% solution with retinoic acid 0.025% or 0.05% along with a corticosteroid (hydrocortisone 1-2.5% or triamcinolone 0.025% twice daily). These preparations should be combined with a sunscreen or sunblock.

Melanex	*3% solution*		
Eloquin Forte	*4% cream*		
Solaquin Forte	*4% cream*	*with sunscreen*	*(Padimate O, Dioxybenzone, oxybenzone)*
Solaquin Forte	*4% get*	*with sunscreen*	*(Padimate O, oxybenzone)*
Eldopaque Forte	*4% cream*	*with tinted sunscreen*	*(iron oxides)*
Viquin Forte	*4% cream*	*with sunscreen*	*(Padimate O, Dioxybenzone, oxybenzone)*
Melquin-3	*3% solution*		
Melquin HP	*4% cream*		

Nuquin HP	*4% cream*	*with sunscreen*	*(Octyl metho-xycinnamate, benzophenone)*
Nuquin HP	*4% gel*	*with sunscreen*	*(dioxybenzone)*
Melpaque HP	*4% cream*	*with tinted sunblock*	*(iron oxides)*

Kojic acid is another tyrosinase inhibitor that prevents formation of new melanin pigment. It is an extract from the fungus *Aspergillus aryzeau*. It may irritate the skin of some patients. Azelez (Allergan Pharmceuticals Inc. Irvine, CA) contains 20% azelaic acid and may be helpful for some patients.

Topical corticosteroids will increase angiogenesis that is a disadvantage after laser resurfacing.

Order of application of skin treaments
Vitamin C products should be applied to a clean well-dried face in the morning. A cleanser and toner are used prior to the Vitamin C. The sun block is followed by make-up. Tretinoins should be applied to a clean well-dried face at bedtime. Treatments for hyperpigmentation (dark pigmented skin blotches) may include kojic acid compounds and hydroquinone in the morning. Your doctor may prescribe this treatment twice a day. It is best to introduce only one treatment regimen at a time to decrease irritation or allergy. One must decide on the priorities of their treatment choices with a physician.

The aging face undergoes various processes that cause sagging of skin and depressions in the face. Specifically, there is decreased skin thickness and elasticity. There is also gradual absorption of subcutaneous tissue and a loosening of the firm attachments of the skin to the underlying layers. These changes result in the gravitational descent of soft tissue with the formation of skin folds along lines of skin adherence where the muscles of facial expression (Friedland JA, Simultaneous laser resurfacing with face lift: A safe alternative for facial rejuvenation. *Aesthetic Surgery Journal* 19:499, 1999). Static wrinkles should be distinguished from dynamic wrinkles. Dynamic wrinkles change with the movement of the muscles underlying the skin of the face that cause facial expression. Such dynamic wrinkles of the overlying skin change in response to contraction of the muscles of facial expression. The dynamic wrinkles are less responsive to blepharoplasty and skin care than static wrinkles which change little with changes in facial expression. Dynamic wrinkles respond well to Botox because of its effect on the underlying musculature. The wrinkles or rhytides whether dynamic or static are virtual linear valleys within the skin due to loss of the collagen. The collage in the dermis is replaced by degenerating so-called elastic tissue. In addition, facial muscle contraction causes wrinkles in the overlying skin. This phenomenon explains the usefulness of Botox that weakens the offending muscle. Your physician is able to work out a skin regimen that is best for you.

Skin care regimens should involve a sun block, a vitamin C to enhance the production of collagen to thicken the underlying dermis of the skin and reduce wrinkles, and a bleaching agent in many patients with pigmentary skin changes that occur during pregnancy or in the menopausal period.

Daily skin care regimens may be enhanced by facial peels. Dr. Mauriello prefers office peels to phenol peels and laser resurfacing. The facial peels are self-neutralizing and, therefore, result in minimal redness, flaking, and downtime. The peels are recommended at monthly intervals for 4 sessions and then repeated every six months as necessary.

Guide to daily home skin care (consult with your physician before embarking on any regimen)

In the Morning—

- Wash
- Toner
- Gel to treatment hyperpigmentation
- Vitamin C topical treatment
- Moisturizer plus sun block

At bedtime—

- Wash
- TONER
- Gel to treat hyperpigmentation
- Tretinoins
- Vitamin C topical treatment
- Moisturizer

Initial skin treatment for pigmentary (irregular skin blotching) skin changes prior to skin rejuvenation with chemical peels
Minimizing sun exposure and the use of sunscreens is necessary at all times. Retinoic acid 0.1% and 4% hydroquinone for 6 weeks are helpful in patients with minimal skin damage due to sun exposure. Only a few patients with minimal pigment changes respond to this simple and nonaggressive treatment. (Baker TM Chemicals and lasers for skin resurfacing. Aesthetic Surgery Journal 1999; 19:325-327).

Alpha hydroxy acids or glycolic acid 30% to 70% are used over several visits in progressively increasing concentrations to abrade the superficial epidermis which has pigment bearing cells (melanocytes) at the basal or lower level of the epidermis. These treatments are suited for younger working women who have only superficial skin changes and neither require nor have the time for more involved procedures.

Non aggressive self neutralizing peels
Peels performed by Dr. Mauriello in his office enhance home care regimens.
Peels may be targeted for patients with dry skin, acne rosacea, garden variety acne, and more darkly pigmented skin in order to avoid unnatural pigmentary changes.

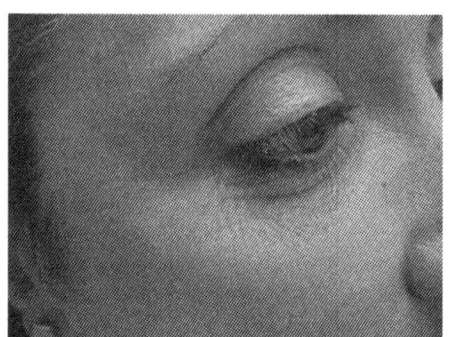 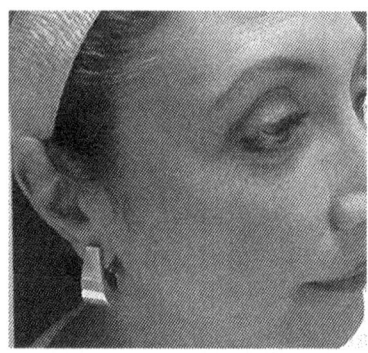

Appearance of skin just
prior to office peel

Appearance immediately
after peel

Patient in photograph above received a 20% trichloroacetic self-neutralizing peel.

In general, psatients note that immediately after the peel, the skin appears smoother and it feels softer. Patients tend to notice changes weeks after the treatment.

AFTER PEEL TREATMENT
- No medications unless prescribed
- Use Cleanser, but no toner, for 3 to 4 days
- Use Sunblock with Moisturizer
    For all other medications, call your physician
- Let stabilize overnight
- Avoid makeup after treatment that day
- Avoid direct sun exposure and excessive heat
- Did not pick at loose skin
- Do not go to a tanning booth
- Avoid electrolysis, collagen, facial waxing or depilatories for five days

FIRST TWO DAYS after office peel
- **No ice**
- **Do not immerse face under shower head**
- **Avoid Jacuzzi, do not swim**
- **Avoid BUFF PUFF**
- **Avoid hair dryer on area treated**

The home care maintenance and office peels improve the quality of the skin and enhance cosmetic eyelid surgery.

Blepharoplasty and skin treatments, including laser resurfacing, chemical peel, and dermabrasion are more effective in removing static wrinkles, but have little, if any, effect on dynamic wrinkles. Botox is helpful in removing both static and dynamic wrinkles as explained earlier in this text.

Aggressive chemical peels and dermabrasion
If patients with dark blotchy pigmentary changes are not improved sufficiently with the above regimen (glycolic acid or hydroquinone), then a trichloroacetic acid (TCA) peel may be helpful. A 35% TCA full face peel is performed in the office in the office without any anesthetic and heals generally in 5-10 days. The redness of the skin lasts 2 to 3 weeks. Superficial lines improve.

The popularity of carbon dioxide and erbium laser skin resurfacing has waned in recent years. There are a host of new lasers introduced at a rapid rate. None to date have been demonstrated to produce results than are better than simple chemical peels including the more aggressive higher concentration trichloroacetic acid peels, phenol peels, or mechanical dermabrasion. Phenol peels and mechanical dermabrasion are particularly helpful in treating raised scars and deep wrinkles, particularly in the mouth area.

Phenol peels require scrupulous technique and considerable experience on the part of the physician to avoid complications. The effect of such aggressive peels that are not self-neutralizing is dependent on the exact solution and its concentration, the length of time it contacts the skin, and the skin type and thickness. The greatest long-term complication of aggressive peels (those that do not self-neutralize) is permanent lack of pigmentation and scarring of the skin. The neck area is particularly prone to scarring because of its lack of hair follicles. The hair follicles provide the epithelium that relines the treated skin and prevents scar tissue from forming.

Suggested Reading

1. Brody JH. Chemical Peeling and Resurfacing. Mosby, St. Louis, Missouri. 1997.

2. Mauriello JA. Editorial commentary on Incisional laser blepharoplasty and laser skin resurfacing, Khan JA in *Unfavorable Results of Eyelid and Lacrimal Surgery Prevention and Management*, Chapter 2, 53-54. Mauriello JA (ed); Butterworth-Heinemann, Boston, Mass, 2000.

GLOSSARY OF COMMON TERMS

atrophy—thinning of a tissue with its normal elements such as fat atrophy of face with aging

blepharon—(Greek) eyelid

blepharoplasty—surgery to repair a defect or correct the eyelid for improve both form and function of the eyelids—cosmetic eyelid surgery, cosmetic eyelid lift
(see definition of "eyelid")

botulinum toxin—Botulinum toxin blocks the nerve impulses that cause a voluntary skeletal muscle to contract and result in wrinkles in the overlying skin. There are several types of botulinum toxin types. Different strains of the bacterium, *Clostridium botulinum,* are used in the preparation of each type of botulinum toxin. Presently, types A and B are commercially available. Botulinum type A is in Botox ® made by Allergan Pharmaceuticals and *Dysport®* by Inamed. Botulinum type B is *Myobloc®*, a product of Elan Pharmaceutical. One unit of Botox ® or Botox ® cosmetic is approximately equivalent to 3-5 Dysport® units and 50-150 Myobloc ® units.

Botulinum toxin is called a "neurotoxin." Botulinum toxin binds to special sites at terminals where the nerve and muscle interface. These terminals are known as motor nerve terminals.

Specifically, botulinum toxin blocks the release of a chemical that causes the muscle to contract. The chemical, known as a neurotransmitter, is called "acetylcholine." Actually, botulinum toxin, the neurotoxin, cleaves to a special protein, the so-called "SNAP-25 protein" that is necessary for the release of the acetylcholine. Without the release of the acetylcholine, the muscle affected by the particular nerve terminal is unable to contract. Botulinum toxin does not inactivate every tiny muscle fiber and, therefore, does not generally lead to complete loss of muscle function. The effect of botulinum toxin is temporary and eventually after 3 to 6 months the muscle contracts.

collagen—fibrous tissue produced by fibroblast cells in the dermis. Fibrous tissue is the framework and scaffold that supports the soft tissues of the body. The bones support the soft tissues which includes the overlying muscles.

canthus—corner of the eye where the upper and lower eyelids meet
> medial (nasal) canthus—corner of the eye by the nose
> lateral (temporal) canthus—corner of the eye by the ear

canthopexy—surgical procedure that supports and usually elevates the inner or outer corners of the eye. A secondary effect is to tighten the skin of the lower eyelid.

canthoplasty- -surgical procedure that involves an actually incision between the upper and lower eyelid in its outer corner. The procedure rearranges the outer corner of the eyelid. A canthoplasty is not generally performed in the inner corner of the eye because any incision would damage the canaliculi or lacrimal drainage system which acts to drain tears from the eye's surface.

commissure—the point where the upper and lower eyelids meet—
> medial (nasal) commissure by the nose
> lateral (temporal commissure) by the ear

conjunctiva—clear layer that extends over sclera. A potential space, the
> subconjunctival space, may fill with blood or fluid due to inflammation as often occurs after surgery. The conjunctiva "joins" the eyelid to the eyeball.

> transconjunctival lower lid blepharoplasty—the incision is bag in through the conjunctiva in the space between the eyelid and eyelid

cornea—outer, front of the eye is an optically clear specialized fibrous tissue (or watch glass) that covers iris (colored part of iris) and is continuous with the white fibrous protective coat of sclera. Its epithelium is non keratinized (does not contain keratin).

crow's feet—wrinkles in the outer corner of the eye. These wrinkles may be static, present when the individual does not smile and dynamic and present upon smiling

dermis—consists of the layers under the overlying superficial lining cells

> The more superficial dermis is the *papillary dermis* which supports the skin while the deeper dermis is the reticular dermis. Chemical peels or carbon dioxide laser resurfacing that destroys the reticular dermis will cause permanent scarring while damage to the papillary dermis promotes new collagen that thickens the skin

edema—fluid that accumulates in tissues after surgery

epidermis—outer layer of cells that line the superficial skin

epithelium—outer layer of cells that line any structure

> The eye surface has conjunctival epithelium and corneal epithelium. These surfaces do not produce keratin since they are mucosal surfaces

erythema—redness is one of the three hallmarks of inflammation, heat, rubor (redness), swelling, and increased temperature due to an increased rate of cellular metabolism. May be due to thermal injury as after carbon dioxide laser or to inflammation induced by the trauma of eyelid surgery

exposure keratitis—exposure of the cornea and drying of the cornea which if untreated may lead to corneal erosion, ulceration, and infection

eyebrow and forehead musculature

> Note: glabella between eyebrows
> corrugator muscle—muscle just above brow that creates frown lines

procerus muscle—muscle that brings brow down and arises from radix (base of nose and inserts into forehead

frontalis muscle—muscle of entire forehead, elevates eyebrow, and creates horizontal furrows eyelid

lower eyelid—from the lower eyelid margin to the inferior orbital rim (bone under the eye)

upper eyelid-from the upper eyelid margin to lower aspect of the eyebrow. Responsible for 75-90% of eyelid closure

eyelid skin—thinnest skin in the body and only placed where muscle is directly underlying the skin with no intervening fat. Elsewhere in the face, such as the cheek, there is fat between the dermis and underlying facial muscles.

fibrous tissue—scar (see definition of "collagen") tissue produced by fibroblasts in order to heal wounds

folds—normal anatomic depressions that may become exaggeratedly deepened with age due to drooping of surrounding tissues and atrophy or thinning of subcutaneous facial fat with age

    nasolabial—fold from corner of nostril to outer corner of mouth

nasojugal—fold between side of nose and cheek (jugal)

upper eyelid—fold of excess skin that overhangs eyelid crease

frown lines—lines or wrinkles in the glabellar area (see definition of "glabella")

glabella—area between the eyebrows where scowl and frown lines appear. This area is often a prime target for Botox cosmetic injections.

hair follicles—are associated with sebaceous glands that express their sebum or oily into the lumen of the hair follicle to serve as an inherent cool cream for the lubrication of the overlying skin.
    The great number of pilosebaceous units distinguish facial from skin outside the face
    The nose and forehead have more sebaceous units than the cheeks or temples

lagophthalmos—inability to close the eyelids which may lead to exposure keratitis (exposure of the cornea and drying of the cornea which if untreated may lead to corneal erosion, ulceration, and infection)

levator muscle—muscle just below the orbital roof (bone above the eye) in the upper eyelid that elevates the upper eyelid.

levator aponeurosis—tendon of the levator muscle which creates the upper eyelid crease *limbus (corneo-scleral limbus)*—circular junction of white sclera and clear cornea where conjunctiva ends and appears to surround iris

malar cheek pad—highest point of cheek or cheek prominence below the eye is composed of thickened fat under skin

melanocyte—pigment cells in the skin responsible for melanin pigment production and the relative lightness (hypopigmented) or darkness (hyerpigmented) of one's skin

    Melanin in the epidermis of the skin, like melanin through-out the body, is produced by a specialized cell termed a "melanocyte."

    The melanin protects the skin surface against ultraviolet light by absorbing UV light

    For this reason, skin cancers do not occur in blacks and rarely in individuals with dark skin

midface—from inferior or lower orbital rim (bone) to mouth

orbit—bone that houses the eyeball and consists of four walls each of which has a corresponding rim or projection of bone that can be felt on the surface of the face below the skin

    medial wall—on the side of the nose (medial orbital rim is not defined since the lacrimal drainage system or sac is located there)

    lateral wall—on the side of the ear (lateral orbital rim is a projection which projects the eye from its side) *roof or superior wall*—above eye (superior orbital rim is covered by the eyebrow)

floor or inferior wall—below eye (inferior orbital rim is below eye)—fat bags prolapse above the inferior orbital rim

pigmentation in the skin—may be due to melanin which causes a tan or collection of blood and its breakdown products after surgery. Blepharoplasty does not remove skin pigmentation or melanin or dark circles in the skin under the eye

plastic surgery—surgery that is characterized by repair of a defect and restoration of apart that affects the form and function of that part.

ptosis-droop
    blepharoptosis—droop of the upper eyelid margin
    brow ptosis—droop of eyebrow
    lash ptosis—downward pointing of the eyelashes over the pupil

reticular dermis—deeper and thicker reticular (net-like structure) layer which when penetrated by the laser during laser resurfacing may result in permanent scarring of the skin

rhytid—wrinkle

sclera—outermost fibrous protective coat of the eye whose front extension is the clear cornea *scleral show*—usually an undesirable result after cosmetic blepharoplasty in which white sclera shows under the limbus of the eye or colored iris to scarring of the lower eyelid

scowl lines—lines or wrinkles in the glabellar area (see definition of "glabella")

stratum corneum—Outermost layer of skin or epidermis is composed of epithelial cells which have a protective role. This horny layer which is produced by the epidermis is composed of keratin. The keratin in the stratum corneum protects against physical damage but also to some extent against sun exposure and is most developed on the palms of the hands and the soles of the feet. The eye surface, like all mucosal surfaces in the body, is not keratinized (does not contain keratin).

tear trough deformity—space under the lower eyelid over the bone of the orbital rim due to gravitational downward sagging of the cheek. The deformity creates shadows under the eyes

0-595-25423-3

www.ingramcontent.com/pod-product-compliance
Lightning Source LLC
Chambersburg PA
CBHW020306290526
45784CB00003B/1385